Praise for *Eve's Blessing*

"Suzannah Weiss is sounding the alarm with the devastating news about women when we are culturally asleep to Eve's curse. Once awake, readers will be greatly relieved and delighted to find the doorway to experience Eve's blessing of pleasure, health, and perhaps even reverence. And that blessing benefits all of us."
  Beverly Dale, founder of the Incarnation Institute for Sex & Faith and author of *Who Told You That You Were Naked? Meditations on the Sexual Body*

"*Eve's Blessing* offers a brilliant, sweeping indictment of a culture – and medical system – that treats women's pain as natural and inevitable and points the way toward a future in which our bodily pleasure and power is a given."
  Maya Dusenbery, author of *Doing Harm: The Truth About How Bad Medicine and Lazy Science Leave Women Dismissed, Misdiagnosed, and Sick*

"Suzannah Weiss has written an incredibly important book – one that is a must-read for women everywhere. And for men. And for the whole of the medical profession. As Suzannah says, 'We've incorrectly diagnosed women as broken when they are showing us what is broken about the world.' *Eve's Blessing* shows what is broken about the world, and how brilliantly it can be mended. You'll come away from this book refuting 'no pain, no gain' forever. Suzannah's

'no pleasure, no gain' is the rallying cry of the future we all want to live in."
Cindy Gallop, founder and CEO of MakeLoveNotPorn

"Another win from Weiss, *Eve's Blessing* is the unrelenting truth-telling serum that our culture needs to take a look at itself and reevaluate the problematic, ignorant, and misogynist norms that still plague our society today. Thank you Weiss for your bravery, critical research, and strong storytelling ability!"
Madame Gandhi, musical artist and activist

"*Eve's Blessing* offers an eye-opening look at women's pain and pleasure. Written in an accessible style, Weiss weaves together history, psychology, science, and personal stories. An empowering and liberating read, this book shatters numerous myths and paves the path to a future with less pain and more pleasure."
Justin Lehmiller, Kinsey Institute, author of *Tell Me What You Want* and host of the Sex and Psychology Podcast

"The message of *Eve's Blessing* is one every woman needs to hear: it is time we expect more pleasure from our lives – and stop expecting pain. Having worked with many women stuck in the mindset that being female means suffering through periods and PMS or not enjoying sex, I know this book will change lives. It raises the bar for how women, sex- and gender-nonconforming people, and men can feel in their bodies – and how we can all support one another to reach our full capacity for comfort and joy."
Laurie Mintz, author of *A Tired Woman's Guide to Passionate Sex* and *Becoming Cliterate: Why Orgasm Equality Matters – And How to Get It*

"Storytelling is powerful, especially when it comes to something as deeply personal as the body, pleasure, pain, and oppression. *Eve's Blessing* offers exactly that – stories that illuminate, heal, and transform, guiding us toward reclaiming the joy and resilience that have always been ours. *Eve's Blessing* weaves personal narratives and cultural insights to challenge the idea that suffering defines the

female body, revealing a path back to joy, resilience, and the pleasure that ought to have always been ours to claim."
Jessica O'Reilly, sex and relationship expert

"*Eve's Blessing* is a gripping, transformative read that weaves the author's personal journey with a profound exploration of history, culture, and the female experience. This book is a reclamation – a call to move beyond pain and shame into power and pleasure, celebrating women's bodies, sexuality, and the full spectrum of their experiences. Suzannah brilliantly exposes how the world has normalized – and even created – women's suffering, from menstrual cycles to sexual experiences and beyond. *Eve's Blessing* is an invitation to break free, awaken your path to pleasure, and recognize its essential role in all aspects of life – including childbirth. Yes, it's possible to have an orgasmic birth too! Prepare to reflect, to challenge what you've been taught, and to shed the layers of shame that have held you back. This book dares you to see what's been hidden in plain sight and embrace the pleasure, power, and liberation that are your birthright. Grab a tissue, grab a notepad, and get ready to reclaim your body – and your joy."
Debra Pascali-Bonaro, director of *Orgasmic Birth: The Best-Kept Secret*, podcast host and international speaker

"*Eve's Blessing* is digestible and gripping, telling a story any woman can relate to. What makes it unique is its interweaving of heartfelt personal journeys, playful deep-dives into history and religion, and indispensable information on health, wellness, and sexuality. This book can help us all create lives – and a world – with more pleasure and less pain."
Tiffany Pham, artist, founder of Mogul and author of *You Are a Mogul: How to Do the Impossible, Do It Yourself, and Do It Now*

"Suzannah Weiss's deep-dive into the worst ramifications of the gender binary – including centuries of pigheaded insistence on normalizing female pain – couldn't be better timed. Holding space for sex and gender diversity as she makes sure to aim her ire where it belongs, this book is a shot across the bow of careless, sexist medical training – because Suzannah has seen the effects of that from the inside – and so much more everyday and state-sponsored misogyny and homo/nb/transphobia. The page decimating the toxic notion of 'no pain, no gain' is worth the price of admission! Voraciously researched, fierce, and clear, this book is a call to arms and a new feminist classic."

Carol Queen, staff sexologist at Good Vibes and director of Center for Sex & Culture

"*Eve's Blessing* is itself a forbidden fruit, full of forbidden knowledge about bodies and desires. Suzannah Weiss skillfully critiques the systems that have perpetuated pain and oppression, and she offers readers a pathway toward pleasure and liberation. Eat the apple."

Eric Sprankle, Minnesota State University, Mankato, and author of *DIY: The Wonderfully Weird History and Science of Masturbation*

"Astoundingly well-researched and illuminating, *Eve's Blessing* is not just a must-have contemporary women's sexual health resource, but a powerful sexual self-help book that uplifts and inspires. Author Suzannah Weiss takes readers on a triumphant journey of sexual healing that will leave you tingling joyously from head to toe."

Hida Viloria, human rights activist and author of *Born Both: An Intersex Life*

"For millennia, women's bodies have been synonymous with pain. Have you had enough? *Eve's Blessing* shows you how to embrace your body's potential for boundless pleasures."

Lisa Wade, Tulane University, author of *American Hookup*

"*Eve's Blessing* is for any woman who has felt her body let her down. Weiss writes with compassion for this experience while illuminating what's available on the other side. The stories are captivating, and the insights gained from them are golden. You won't be able to put this book down."

Maitland Ward, actress and model

Eve's Blessing

Sisterhood and siblinghood enabled me to birth this book in pleasure, not in painful toil. So I dedicate this book to the cursed who blessed me. To the mysteriously ill, the frigid lovers, moody bitches, negative Nancies, nervous Nellies, and borderline babes. Those with blood coming out of their wherever, and those who don't bleed but are still part of the siblinghood.

Eve's Blessing
Uncovering the Lost Pleasure Behind Female Pain

SUZANNAH WEISS

polity

Copyright © Suzannah Weiss 2025

The right of Suzannah Weiss to be identified as Author of this Work has been asserted in accordance with the UK Copyright, Designs and Patents Act 1988.

First published in 2025 by Polity Press

Polity Press
65 Bridge Street
Cambridge CB2 1UR, UK

Polity Press
111 River Street
Hoboken, NJ 07030, USA

All rights reserved. Except for the quotation of short passages for the purpose of criticism and review, no part of this publication may be reproduced, stored in a retrieval system or transmitted, in any form or by any means, electronic, mechanical, photocopying, recording or otherwise, without the prior permission of the publisher.

ISBN-13: 978-1-5095-6616-7
ISBN-13: 978-1-5095-6617-4 (pb)

A catalogue record for this book is available from the British Library.

Library of Congress Control Number: 2024952278

Typeset in 11 on 14pt Warnock Pro
by Fakenham Prepress Solutions, Fakenham, Norfolk NR21 8NL
Printed and bound in Great Britain by CPI Group (UK) Ltd, Croydon

The publisher has used its best endeavours to ensure that the URLs for external websites referred to in this book are correct and active at the time of going to press. However, the publisher has no responsibility for the websites and can make no guarantee that a site will remain live or that the content is or will remain appropriate.

Every effort has been made to trace all copyright holders, but if any have been overlooked the publisher will be pleased to include any necessary credits in any subsequent reprint or edition.

For further information on Polity, visit our website:
politybooks.com

Contents

Content Note and Disclaimer — vii

Introduction — 1

Part I: The Fall — 9

1. Curses Were Meant to Be Broken — 13
2. Women's Natural Defectiveness and Other Greek Myths — 27
3. From Stained Sheets to White Houses: The Painful Price of Pleasure — 37
4. Men's Bodies Are from Mars, Women's Are from Venus — 48
5. How the Female Orgasm Became Elusive — 59
6. PMS, from "a Raging Animal" to "Blood Coming Out of Her Wherever" — 74
7. The Institutionalization of Sorrowful Childbirth — 87
8. Trauma: An Assault on the Body — 103
9. Sexy But Not Sexual — 117

Part II: Paradise Gained — 127

10 Womanhood Is Not an Illness — 129
11 Period Pleasure — 139
12 No Pleasure, No Gain — 149
13 In Joy Thou Shalt Bring Forth Children — 157
14 I Will Greatly Multiply Thy Orgasms — 168
15 Living Life Orgasmically — 177
Epilogue: Original Virtue — 193

Resource List — 197
Notes — 201

Content Note and Disclaimer

This book contains stories involving medical and sexual trauma. If you're sensitive to medical trauma, I'd recommend skipping chapter 7 or reading it in a safe space where you can access support. If you're sensitive to sexual trauma, I'd recommend the same for chapter 8.

Eve's Blessing shares several people's chronic illness journeys, including my own. A few of these stories describe medical treatments, some conventional and others alternative. This book is not medical advice. I'm not advocating specific interventions but giving people a platform to share, in their own words and on their own terms, how they've learned to enjoy their bodies in a world working against their thriving. I recommend you ask a healthcare provider about anything shared that resonates with you, and see the resource list at the end for help.

Lastly, this book is less a critique of the Bible than a reimagining of it – one that honors all religions' core teaching of uplifting the downtrodden. So whatever your religious background – or lack thereof – please stick around. There may be something here for you to sink your teeth into.

Introduction

One night at sleepaway camp, ten-year-old me lay in a bunk bed playing Mad Libs with my cabin-mates. From the other side of the cramped wooden room, one girl read out a prompt to describe "a bad day." Another suggested, "the day before your period!"

"What's a period?" I asked.

"It's when your thing bleeds and you grow hair there," she replied matter-of-factly, if not totally correctly. At the time, I didn't know better. I was horrified to learn this bad day was in my future – and even more terrified to later realize it was not just a day. In health class that fall, I received more education about periods – and more miseducation. Warnings about cramps, PMS, and unplanned pregnancy dominated the female discussion. Then came the male lesson, which covered phenomena like erections and wet dreams that were physically, if not always psychologically, pleasurable.

As I wandered through my school's moss green carpeted hallways, I fantasized that by some feat of magic, I could become a boy. That I could avoid the agonizing puberty awaiting girls. The expectation of female pain continued from high school whispers about first-time sex into my twenties and thirties, when healthcare providers shrugged off my sexual struggles and chronic illness symptoms. The message was clear: Women were cursed. Penises – conflated with men in my early education – were simple and easy and happy. Vulvas, vaginas, and uteruses were tricky, problem-prone, and burdensome.

Nurturing a Better Nature

Philosophers, theologians, and scientists alike have dubbed women deficient since the dawn of Western civilization, and the belief in women's physical inferiority lingers. It lingers in doctors' dismissal of women's health complaints. It lingers in jokes about women's premenstrual incompetence. It lingers in the very notion that men and women are the only people to exist – and exist as biological opposites. It lingers in the expectation that menstruation should hurt, that sex should hurt, that childbirth should hurt, that being a woman should hurt.

Today, actresses from Zooey Deschanel in *New Girl* to Natalie Portman in *No Strings Attached* are seen doubled over in pain and unable to function during their periods. Losing your virginity is dubbed "popping your cherry." Articles lament the "elusive female orgasm." The underlying assumptions are couched in biological arguments about the evolutionary role of PMS, the hymen, and anorgasmia. On the surface, statistics appear to support these hypotheses. Up to 91% of women suffer from period pain.[1] One in thirteen currently experience pain during sex.[2] Between 5 and 10% of women have never had an orgasm.[3] Women report poorer physical health than men and are more often diagnosed with chronic pain, anxiety, and depression.[4] Yet nothing about these disparities is inevitable. It is our continued reliance on ancient theories about the female body – not the body itself – that makes womanhood synonymous with pain. Media, politics, science, and medicine can make the fruits of oppression appear natural, neglecting that nurture shapes nature. That's exactly what's been done with women's pain and pleasurelessness. The curse is not womanhood; it's misogyny. It is a cultural curse we are under.

Imparting the stories of women and gender-diverse people who alchemized pain into pleasure, this book aims to give readers a new perception of their bodies – one that challenges the bleak messages around them. One that simultaneously acknowledges their pain and their capacity to move beyond it. One that proves we need not surmount our biology to attain equality. It's inequality that flies in the face of our design. As I paint this large-scale picture, you'll follow my own path from pain to pleasure – one full of sexual exploration, spiritual growth, and trying times as I mourned the curse seemingly on me and all women, then uncovered the blessings behind it.

Through my own transformation, I realized our views of women's bodies have enormous stakes. If we deem some gender inequalities innate simply because they're physiological – neglecting how inequality shapes physiology – societal problems from the orgasm gap to the female chronic illness epidemic seem like nature taking its course rather than injustices to be rectified. And so nobody takes a stand against them. More than that, women's sense of confidence and competence is under siege. When women learn they are built for less pleasure and more pain than men, they accept lives where they experience just that. Feeling unequal on a biological level, they carry themselves with an air of inferiority. It follows them to work, into their relationships, everywhere. No matter how many feminists challenge stereotypes about women's mental unfitness, the denigration of our physical and sexual selves continues to tarnish our views of gender in every arena.

The Path from Paradise to Pain ... and Back

As a child, I was flooded with inaccurate, decontextualized, and downright frightening information about my body. I missed out on years I could have spent enjoying (or at least working toward) radiant health, relishing life-affirming sexual connections, and celebrating my body rather than feeling ashamed of it. But in the end, I found the resources to turn things around. Through the support of women around me, I learned to advocate for my right to respect from doctors, attention from sexual partners, and a life that's not just comfortable but joyful. Some are denied these opportunities their whole lives due to gender, race, class, and ability barriers. Nobody teaches them anything other than that it is normal, acceptable, to suffer and forgo pleasure. That period pain, PMS, and painful sex are inevitable. That female arousal is finicky. That women are innately inferior. Yet when we dismantle this myth, a sense of innate equality takes its place. And with this sense of innate biological equality, women feel justified in fighting for social equality.

I'll begin *Eve's Blessing* by examining where the notion of female defectiveness comes from, starting with the Greek philosophers' juxtapositions between the sexes and the Bible's punishment of Eve, then making my way through history, from the superstitious virginity tests of medieval times to the early modern era's marriage manuals. I'll document how the Enlightenment-age gendering of bodies makes healthcare an uphill battle for sex and gender-diverse people, how Victorian purity ideals spawned a view of women as passionless, and how two murderers shaped popular discourse around PMS. These ideologies' repercussions reverberate through hospitals and bedrooms alike, compounded by modern injustices like rape culture, media sexualization, and medical bias that keep women from enjoying their anatomy. We've incorrectly diagnosed women as broken when they're showing us what's broken about the world.

Nobody knows this better than those who have dealt with pain and pleasurelessness themselves – and been told by peers and professionals alike that their complaints are invalid. I have spoken to many such people and will weave them into the following chapters, showing how their stories have unfolded within a broader cultural crisis. Drawing on my expertise as a sexologist, psychotherapist, and birth doula while quoting experts from doctors to theologians, I'll unveil the epidemic of female pain and pleasurelessness as symptomatic of a sick society. I'll show how toxic consumerism contributes to period pain, how under-researched, underdiagnosed gynecological conditions cause painful sex, and how sexual violence spawns anxiety, depression, and chronic pain. Women struggling with their bodies are canaries in the coalmine, alerting us to the stress, disconnection, and exploitation endemic to Western culture. And certain populations like women of color and gender-diverse people are particularly vulnerable. While the ideas I'm critiquing conflate women and wombs – and I'll sometimes do so for linguistic simplicity – I'll examine how they can affect anyone who has a vulva, uterus, or female identity. In fact, the same stereotypes that spawn assumptions about female inferiority also erase those outside the gender binary. I'll demonstrate how this plays out using interviews with intersex, two-spirit, trans, and non-binary people abused and neglected by the healthcare system.

Welcome to a New Womanhood

Despite the heavy subject matter, this book ends on a triumphant note, documenting how people are creating new bodily realities for themselves and others. I'll chronicle how the early chapters' characters realized their challenges reflected underlying problems – then solved them. Readers will find out how one woman learned her "normal" period pain stemmed from a common yet poorly grasped illness, how another invented a device to treat painful intercourse, and how one discovered her orgasmic capacity at a masturbation workshop. Though the last few millennia have devised a dismal definition of womanhood, a new narrative of our bodies is emerging, thanks to women like these. Forward-looking healthcare providers and entrepreneurs are combating period pain and PMS. Activists, artists, and academics are spreading awareness of what women need in bed – and giving them the confidence to attain it. Doulas and midwives are reclaiming childbirth as a positive experience. Sex educators are showing women their pleasure potential goes beyond what they imagined. Collectively, we are coming to see that vulvas, vaginas, and uteruses are not curses. They are blessings.

None of this means women's pain is not real. I myself know that it is. My own path to pleasure was paved with pain: years of sexual numbness, compromised mental health, and a series of physical symptoms that went on for years like some sick joke. But the real sickness of the joke lay in its masking of the truth: that my body was functioning perfectly. It was launching a healthy response to an unhealthy world. Once you put down this book, you will be able to imagine a world that's well. A world where women expect periods, first-time sex, and other "painful" experiences to be painless, expect sex to be pleasurable, and expect their bodies to be pleasant places to reside in. Though there are real obstacles to this goal right now, it will become clear that these impediments are cultural and therefore changeable. And in changing the culture, we can change our relationship to our bodies and ourselves. We can rewrite the ages-old script that says we must prove ourselves worthy of joy.

Many of us grew up believing we deserve displeasure. Whether or not we were raised religiously, Eve's apple is baked into the culture we consume. We live under the subtle influence of a punishing God, learning that gain is only possible through pain. We are taught that we must work for the sustenance we earn, that hardship is the dues we pay for thriving. That too much fun is merely an indulgence. But what if pleasure were not a forbidden fruit? What if Adam and Eve's sensuality and curiosity were worthy of reward? What if God's so-called punishment – Eve must give birth in sorrow – is a metaphor for misogyny's impact on our bodies? What if we have what it takes to return to paradise, and the curse was simply a gripping plot twist, a hurdle to overcome? And what if Adam's curse – he must support himself through painful toil – was set up to be unwound along with Eve's? As we challenge ideals of arduous labor – reproductive and economic – that are harming everyone's health, we can rediscover that we were all born blessed.

My desire to write this book stems from the liberation I experienced in shattering myths about women's bodies in my own wellness journey – and finding a delightful amount of pleasure where I expected pain. I've sprinkled in my own story to create a thread you can follow from beginning to end, making myself a guide through history, present times, and the lives of people who achieved victories for their health and sexuality. After savoring such victories myself, I believe the first step toward helping others attain the same is teaching them it's possible. Discomfort and dissatisfaction aren't natural after all. In fact, there's an endless well of joy behind our sorrow, just waiting to be unlocked. That's something I wish I'd been taught in school – and something we can all teach our children if we want them to live pleasurable, pain-free lives.

Part I

The Fall

Women are born with pain built in. It's our physical destiny: period pains, sore boobs, childbirth, you know. We carry it within ourselves throughout our lives. Men don't.

— Fleabag[1]

Countless women take this as a given, rarely questioning the pain that plagues them. When Abby developed debilitating period cramps as a preteen, she didn't think to tell her doctor. Nor did Amanda when sex hurt, not just the first time but many times after. Celia mentioned her menstrual pain to doctors, but they simply told her to lose weight. Meg was on an emotional rollercoaster the week before her period, for which she only knew to pop Midol. When Tara told her gynecologist about the burning sensations sex caused her, he advised her to have a glass of wine. While Sarah was in the ER with severe constipation, a doctor reassured her this was "quite normal" since "51% of women complain of constipation."[2] And when America asked her urologist what treatment was available for her excruciating bladder illness, he replied, "none."

Debra hid in a maternity ward bathroom during labor to escape staff who pushed medications on her. When Tanisha developed bladder spasms after childbirth, a staff member looked on, detached, declaring, "You would make an interesting paper." Hida's doctors harped on irrelevant questions like "do you feel more like a man or a woman?" and "has your clitoris always been this big?" Ed couldn't get his PCOS treated until a gender identity clinic certified it was in his "psychiatric best interests." Whenever Kuya had to check "male" or "female" on a medical form, it reminded them their culture, which has more than two genders, wasn't valued. Up until her forties, Sammi had never had an orgasm; she blamed her small clitoris. Kaytlin blamed her difficulty orgasming with partners on the female body's complexity.

Such struggles are valorized as an honor of womanhood, as if our strength stemmed from enduring pain – usually for the sake of children or partners. They are brushed off for those outside the gender binary, as if their bodies were broken to begin with. At best, they're deemed yet another case of "life isn't fair." Yet these problems' commonality does not make them normal or natural. While the status quo seems to paint a grim picture of the female body, the picture it paints is actually of Western culture. Women have spent millennia abused and discriminated against, and the price has been their physical health, comfort, and pleasure. Though patriarchy wants us to forget, our bodies remember. But the memories stored in our cells can be unwound and shed – and that's already happening.

The idea that women and gender-diverse people's lives could be as physically enjoyable as men's was perhaps true only in theory a few years ago. Between medicine's neglect for marginalized people and the political, cultural, and economic obstacles keeping us sick and unhappy, society was not set up for it. But today, women are forging their own paths out of pain that others can now travel – and what they're finding on the other side is pleasure. They're fighting to be heard in medical settings and spreading awareness of under-discussed health issues. They're inventing their own solutions to painful periods and sex. And they're having lots of orgasms – multiple orgasms, varied kinds of orgasms, and even orgasmic births. Why does it seem, then, that women are designed to endure less pleasant lives than men? Answering this question requires a journey back in time.

Chapter 1

Curses Were Meant to Be Broken

This story begins at its destination – paradise – with two people like you and me. You might've heard this part. Adam and Eve were luxuriating in the Garden of Eden, naked and unashamed, when a serpent made a scandalous suggestion: that Eve eat from the tree of knowledge of good and evil, something God forbade. She offered Adam some fruit too, and suddenly, they grew aware they were naked. In response, a displeased God told Eve: "I will make your pains in childbearing very severe; with painful labor you will give birth to children." The first woman, who once lived in comfort, was now embarrassed of her body and at odds with it. The first man did not fare well either; he was told: "Cursed is the ground because of you; through painful toil you will eat food from it."[1] Both stood on cursed ground. The soil that once sprouted plentiful nourishment would require human strain to support survival. Both men and women, in their own ways, would spend their days in labor. In pain.

The Fall from Equality to Oppression

When I revisit this tale, I think of a passage from *Sex at Dawn*, an anthropological account of human sexuality. Authors Christopher Ryan and Cacilda Jethá write that humanity's true "fall" was not from a garden but from a "jungle, forest, wild seashore, open savanna, [or] wind-blown tundra." These prehistoric environments were home to nomadic hunter-gatherers who enjoyed privileges Adam and Eve did: "Their world provided what they needed: food, shelter, and companionship." The small tribes were cooperative by necessity, they could build huts in minutes, meals were shared, and the pursuit of sexual pleasure – including women's – was permitted. Then, as agriculture sprung up globally around 10,000 BC, the "low-stress, high-pleasure life of foragers" was usurped by "the dawn-to-dusk toil of a farmer." Ryan and Jethá theorize that "the story of the fall gives narrative structure to the traumatic transition from the take-it-where-you-find-it hunter-gatherer existence to the arduous struggle of agriculturalists."[2] The plentiful Garden of Eden's transformation into a stubborn field mirrors humanity's move from forests full of fruits to land they had to fight to extract crops from.

That was Adam's curse, but it led to Eve's. Humanity's transition from cooperative, egalitarian tribes to civilizations revolving around property set the stage for women to be property. Some anthropologists pinpoint the advent of agriculture as patriarchy's harbinger.[3] The plow encouraged gendered divisions of labor, with men seen as fit for plowing fields while women stayed home. Even today, societies descending from plow farmers display more gender disparities in work and politics.[4] But something deeper was happening. Since agrarians stayed in one place and built houses, they formed nuclear family units. To track which children belonged to which fathers – and pass down real estate, crops, and animals accordingly – they restricted women's sexuality and freedom. Without female monogamy, family lines were hard to trace.[5] And so childbearing came under collective control, leading women to indeed bring forth children in pain. Emotional pain. Their procreation faced scrutiny; their autonomy was taken away. They were scorned for not having children or for having them outside marriage. Eve's desire became shameful. She grew to recognize her nakedness. To restrain her corporeality, her passion, her power.

The apple didn't fall far from the tree, and it was a poisonous one.[6] While the world may have never been pure paradise, the fall from foraging to farming introduced new forms of pain: women's painful labor and men's painful toil. The parallel between Genesis and human history is more direct with Adam's curse – men began working to eat – but the transition affected women just as much. It took them from equality and communal resource sharing to patriarchy and, eventually, capitalism. And patriarchy and capitalism have real, direct effects on women's health and happiness. Women's bodies bear the brunt of the fall, not just when giving birth but throughout their lives.

The burden women bear is compounded by the very belief that they are cursed – in more than one way. Though God's curse on Eve most clearly references childbirth, periods are also called "the curse" in some religious communities.[7] Not just Judeo-Christian ones. Eleven percent of women in Pakistan consider menstruation God's way of punishing womankind, and 12% of girls in India see it as a disease or curse from God.[8] The notion of the curse prevails in pop culture and everyday lingo. In the 1976 film *Carrie*, the protagonist's mother exclaims upon her first period: "The Lord visited Eve with the curse, and the curse was the curse of blood. Oh, Lord! Help this sinning woman see the sin of her days and ways. Show her that if she had remained sinless, this curse of blood would never have come on her!"[9] A 1948 study identified "curse" as the most common American period euphemism, and another from 1963 documented "curse," "sickness," and "unwell."[10] Even in 1994, nearly half of women in an Oregon study had used or heard the term "curse" for menstruation.[11] Modern women are still believed to be paying for Eve's sin. Even many who don't deem periods a literal curse expect them to feel like one.

Period Pain: Normal or Normalized?

When Abby Norman got her first period at age twelve and a half, she was spending Thanksgiving with her family. But she didn't enjoy much time with them, as she passed the whole day in the bathroom with cramps, diarrhea, nausea, and thigh pain. "I thought I was bleeding so much because it was my first period, but then they were always like that," she recalls. "I always felt sick and had a lot of pain. I've never had a period that wasn't painful. But I thought that was normal, and I never knew anything different."

Celia similarly had "sickeningly unbearable" periods since age thirteen. "I vividly remember being in class and having to beg for a pain reliever," she says. "I went to an all-girls' high school, and thankfully, my mom was also a teacher. So she approved it, and then I had to just lay down in the nurse's office until they kicked in. Usually, what would happen is the pain was so intense that by the time it was over, I was just so exhausted and I would fall asleep." Yet this didn't strike her as unusual. "As I got older and the pain got worse and more frequent, it continued," she recounts. "Pain during sex? Oh yeah, that's just a position that hurts. Everyone has that. Cramping after orgasm? Oh yeah, that's normal, everyone has that." Celia can't remember where she learned this; she says "it's always been there. Always." But Abby can point to a few sources: "Pretty much every conversation I had with an older woman – or any book I read – said that cramps were normal and that I just had to put up with it. Every time someone got their period in a TV show or movie, it was always depicted that way."

Menstrual pain is portrayed on screen for humor, masking its serious nature. In the sitcom *New Girl*, Zooey Deschanel's character Jess declares, "It feels like a fat man is sitting on my uterus."[12] Such bleak depictions of menstruation ring true for many, but largely because of this very normalization. It's a self-perpetuating cycle: Since women and their doctors don't search for solutions to their pain, they suffer through it for years – sometimes for life. "Doctors certainly never seemed surprised that my periods hurt," says Abby. "They also didn't usually seem to bat an eye if I said I had pelvic pain at other times during my cycle." It took her seven years to be diagnosed with endometriosis, a condition where tissue similar to the uterine lining grows outside the uterus. And she considers herself one of the "lucky ones": Endometriosis takes ten years to diagnose on average.[13] Black women with this illness have an even harder time getting diagnosed; doctors assume they have pelvic inflammatory disease, which is associated with sexually transmitted infections.[14]

For Celia, it was not just sexism and racism but fatphobia that kept her from a diagnosis for twenty-eight years. When she confided in healthcare providers about her painful periods and sex, she was told "losing weight will help" so many times she just dropped it. "I kind of shut myself off from asking about these things, both out of shame and out of the fact that I just didn't want to be told again that I could somehow reverse this pain with weight loss," she says. Doctors also made remarks about her facial hair, which felt like subtle jabs at her Lebanese heritage. Of course, when she lost weight, it didn't alleviate the pain at all. "It's hard when you've been dismissed for so long to keep bringing it up," Celia says. "You just start to internalize that and think you are being dramatic; it must be normal because no one really seems to think it's a big deal or an actual problem."

Period pain *appears* normal. Studies have found that primary dysmenorrhea – menstrual pain unattributed to any illness – occurs in 60–91% of women globally.[15] But given the prevalence of undiagnosed illnesses, many such women may have *secondary* dysmenorrhea – menstrual pain stemming from underlying health conditions.[16] Many ailments that make periods unbearable, including endometriosis, fibroids, polycystic ovary syndrome (PCOS), and adenomyosis, go untreated for years because period pain is so normalized. Here we have a feedback loop: The sheer number of people living with these conditions makes their symptoms appear common and therefore normal, causing even more people to dismiss their own symptoms and live with them. But normal and common are not the same – and even commonplace pain reflects underlying problems. The issue is, many problems behind menstrual pain are not the type doctors are trained to diagnose. They are manifestations of larger-scale issues like misogyny and poverty. They are the fruits of the fall.

A Cultural Curse

Nicole endured debilitating period cramps for fifteen years and menstrual migraines for almost as long. They made her "feel like not being alive." In the absence of a diagnosis, her doctor presented painkillers and birth control as her only options. "They told me I'd have this condition for life and it was unfortunate, but nothing could be done," she remembers. This is a popular prognosis, as primary dysmenorrhea's causes are unclear. Yet research is beginning to point toward a confluence of environmental, nutritional, chemical, and cultural factors that lurk, barely detectable, behind "normal" period pain.

During menstruation, lipid compounds in the body called prostaglandins make the uterus contract. Prostaglandin levels drop from the beginning to the end of your period, which is why people tend to feel more pain on their first few days of bleeding. The American College of Obstetricians and Gynecologists cites prostaglandins as the cause of primary dysmenorrhea.[17] However, many medical professionals agree it is not ordinary prostaglandin activity but prostaglandin *imbalances* that lead to pain, says Mary Lou Ballweg, president of the Endometriosis Association. A 2015 paper in *Human Reproduction Update*, for instance, reads that "the most widely accepted explanation for the pathogenesis of primary dysmenorrhea is the overproduction of uterine PGs [prostaglandins]."[18] When too many prostaglandins are released, this causes inflammation, an immune system response involving temperature increase, blood flow changes, pain, and/or swelling.[19] High prostaglandin levels have been found in women with primary dysmenorrhea and endometriosis, and drugs that reduce prostaglandin production also reduce menstrual pain.[20] A 2021 American Academy of Family Physicians paper states that primary dysmenorrhea is "mediated by elevated prostaglandin and leukotriene levels"; leukotrienes are also inflammatory.[21] While some inflammation is necessary for the uterus to push out blood, the sheer prevalence of period pain indicates that many of our bodies are overly inflamed. And this excess of inflammation, prostaglandins, and pain reflects some of society's biggest injustices.

One such injustice is businesses' lack of care for consumers, a lingering fragment of the fall from cooperative communities to a trade-based economy. A fall that has continued as large corporations have gained power. Today, many products contain ingredients that create hormonal dysregulation over time. "Our modern world is overwhelmed by chemicals which have hormonal properties," Ballweg explains. "They often accumulate in our bodies, taking over the role of our natural hormones and creating havoc. For example, our work showed that dioxins, often called the most toxic chemical ever produced by man, inactivate progesterone receptors that are needed for a healthy uterus and healthy menstruation." The World Health Organization recognizes the role of dioxins – toxic byproducts of paper bleaching – in reproductive illness, immune system damage, and cancer.[22] Studies have linked dioxins with disrupted hormone signaling and endometriosis.[23] Yet dioxins are found in tampons, pads, and, more frequently, food, mainly due to industrial processing.[24]

Dioxins are but one type of hormone-disrupting chemical. Xenoestrogens – estrogen-mimicking compounds also linked to hormonal imbalances – are present in skincare products, Tupperware, plastic water bottles, pesticides, nail polish, and makeup.[25] Women are the primary users of such products, thanks to gendered advertising and beauty norms. Phthalates and parabens, two types of xenoestrogens, have been found in menstrual supplies as well.[26] And, sure enough, those with higher xenoestrogen exposure report more period pain.[27] "The available information strongly indicates that environmental exposure to EDCs [endocrine-disrupting chemicals] such as PCBs, dioxins, BPA, and phthalates individually or collectively contribute to the pathophysiology of endometriosis," reads a Texas A&M University paper.[28] This issue is well-established enough that certain hormone disruptors like parabens are banned in the European Union – but still not in the US, which prioritizes manufacturers' interests.[29]

The standard Western diet – one dominated by refined sugars, refined oils, and ultra-processed foods but low on whole foods – may also play a role in menstrual pain. For one Georgetown University study, when thirty-three American women adopted a vegetarian diet free from added oils, their menstrual pain decreased within two cycles.[30] A larger study in Iran found that women with diets centered on sugar, caffeine, salty snacks, and added fats were over four times as likely to experience moderate menstrual pain as those who ate mainly vegetables, fruits, legumes, and dairy.[31] And a 258-woman study in Spain linked menstrual pain with soda and meat consumption.[32] The overarching theme of this research, according to a Rutgers University meta-analysis, is that since inflammation causes period pain, inflammatory diets exacerbate it.[33] "I found diets high in inflammatory foods such as animal meats, oil, sugars, salts, and coffee contribute to an increased risk of pain," the review's author Serah Sannoh told CNN. "People with diets high in omega-6 fatty acids, specifically those derived from animal-based products, have a higher presence of arachidonic acid in the body, which increases the amount of pro-inflammatory prostaglandins that help the uterus contract."[34]

This is not to demonize fats or any food group. In fact, omega-3 fatty acids like those in fish and nuts are anti-inflammatory and may reduce menstrual pain.[35] The issue is not that some enjoy sugar or fats, which can be part of a healthy diet. The real issue is Adam's curse: that we eat through "painful toil." That quality nourishment is not readily available. Economic inequality leaves people reliant on foods cheap to manufacture and acquire, which may not only contain inflammatory ingredients but lack nutrients.[36] Menstrual pain has been linked to diets deficient in fruit, omega-3s, protein, and vitamins D and B12, which can result from poverty, dieting, and disordered eating.[37] Industrialization has amplified agriculture's downfalls, with "big food" favoring practices that harm workers, animals, the environment, and our bodies.[38] Modern farming conventions contribute to malnutrition and consumption of deleterious chemicals. Deforestation depletes soil of nutrients, pesticides throw off hormones and disrupt the menstrual cycle, and factory-farmed animals are fed diets that promote inflammation and omega-6/omega-3 imbalances in human consumers.[39]

Eve's descendants are suffering for Adam's curse in more ways than that. We suffer from a work-centered culture that causes chronic stress we didn't evolve to sustain. People are laboring their days away to meet the demands of breadwinning and corporate-ladder-climbing. This affects our bodies: High levels of the stress hormone cortisol throw off women's sex hormones.[40] Research has linked period pain with stress, lack of job control, and employment insecurity.[41] Women with high stress levels are twice as likely as those with low stress to experience menstrual pain.[42] Period pain has also been linked to sleep deprivation and sedentary lifestyles – common results of juggling work and parenting in disconnected societies.[43] Isolation, burnout, poor medical care, toxic products, a lack of time or money to eat well ... these are things many accept as part of modern life when they are hurting women's health – and all our health. That's the real curse.

Feeling the World's Pain

There's a haunting symbolism to this phenomenon. Our bodies are in pain, a signal something's wrong, because something is wrong – with the world around us. Chemical exposure, nutritional imbalances, and long work weeks may not create health problems by themselves. But over time, combined, and on the macro scale, these everyday aspects of our lives have an impact. And there's not much help available for those affected by them. Issues like diet, lifestyle, environmental sensitivities, and stress are relegated to alternative medicine, which isn't usually covered by US insurance.[44] The medical establishment doesn't prioritize women's well-being enough to address our pain unless it reaches extreme levels, and sometimes even when it does. We need a "real" problem to receive real treatment, and period pain is not considered one.

And so, there's that familiar feedback loop: The idea that women are cursed leads them to feel cursed. The treatment of female pain as normal leads women down the path of pain.

Then our pain is presented as evidence that we are indeed cursed, designed for discomfort. Awareness of these issues is hindered by denial that those with menstrual pain are unwell or in need. Menstruation, after all, is itself supposedly an illness. Leviticus calls it a "sickness" or "disease."[45] This made more sense long ago, when menstruation could actually spread disease due to inadequate hygiene.[46] Yet today, we continue to equate it with compromised well-being. So when it does compromise people's well-being, it seems normal. Modern-day medicine is still shaped by ancient mores that deem illness an intrinsic part of womanhood.

Yet what the Old Testament says is true: Men and women *do*, each in their own ways, labor in pain. Menstruation *is* experienced like an illness by many. But we need not conclude that women are destined for doom or facing a divine being's wrath. Instead, perhaps the "curse" the Bible describes was a forecast for humanity's trajectory – a trajectory that need not continue. Perhaps it was set up to be unwound.[47] Maybe it wasn't a punishment. Maybe it was not even a curse. God's declarations to Eve never included the word "curse." He only cursed the serpent and the ground below Adam.[48] If there is a curse on women's bodies, it is human-made. But if any deity enabled it, perhaps that's because the curse itself is a blessing. Perhaps the adventure of unwinding it is better than being blessed from beginning to end. Perhaps it's giving us exactly what Adam and Eve sought: knowledge of good and evil. Through pain, we can get intimate with pleasure. Eve was born blessed, but she chose an extra blessing: the journey of remembering her blessedness in a world that forgot it. Every story, after all, needs a conflict before reaching a satisfying resolution. The history of humanity is no different. The problem isn't Genesis; it's the forgetting that it was only a genesis. It's the false assumption that Eve's story is over. It is just beginning. We are living it now.

The Body of a Second-Class Citizen

Aimee Eyvazzadeh, an endocrinologist in the California Bay Area, sees patients who have undergone hysterosalpingographies (HSGs) – X-ray procedures where a tube in the uterus diagnoses fertility issues. This is "described online and by women everywhere as one of the most painful procedures they've ever had," Eyvazzadeh told me over email. She offers Valium and Tylenol with codeine when she performs HSGs herself, but 99% of her patients who got them elsewhere received no pain meds whatsoever. They were told, "You're a woman. You want to be pregnant, don't you? How do you think that's going to feel? You better get used to it now," she said. "I think that society has created this notion that women should suffer because we are women." When I asked her where this notion comes from, she replied the next morning:

> I went to bed thinking about this one. But I woke up thinking of just one word or sentence: second-class citizens. Women have historically been seen as second-class citizens. Our rights have been restricted. We are viewed still in most nations as not equal to men. And as a result, our access to adequate healthcare is affected.

This is why women's pain appears normal. Not because of our biology, but because women are second-class citizens. If we look beyond our oppression and consider the facts, the illusion of "normal" pain dissolves. Severe menstrual pain occurs in only 12–14% of women worldwide – which could be entirely accounted for by the large cohort with undiagnosed illnesses.[49] One in ten women worldwide has endometriosis, 7% have been diagnosed with uterine tumors called fibroids, and one in ten has a hormonal disorder called polycystic ovary syndrome.[50] What we've deemed a natural part of being female may actually be a "natural" part of being sick in a world unable to help you.

"If someone is experiencing pain so severe and lasting that they are missing school or work, I don't think that could ever be called normal by any reasonable medical or social standard," says Abby. Ballweg doesn't think *any* pain is normal. Pain is a sign that something's off, she points out; it drives us to take action to heal. Yet when such a signal comes from our uteruses, we are silenced as we try to heed it. Menstruation is "a routine monthly function," Ballweg says. "If a routine function such as bowel movements were to be consistently painful, it would not be considered normal. It's only because of the taboo and stigma and shame that have surrounded menstruation that people have allowed this myth to develop. Many other types of health problems are common – ED, enlarged prostate in older men – but not considered normal." If period pain were not a signal something was wrong, living with it would have no negative consequences. But neglecting the menstrual cycle's messages has dire consequences. When we brush off our pain, it escalates into problems no one would call ordinary. The longer menstrual pain goes untreated, the more likely it is to cause other conditions like pelvic floor dysfunction, says Iris Orbuch, a gynecologist specializing in endometriosis. And whatever caused it in the first place remains unaddressed. Even primary dysmenorrhea has been linked to increased pain sensitivity all month long – not just while bleeding – which could explain why it's a risk factor for the neurological pain condition fibromyalgia.[51] As Abby puts it:

> Having my body endure all of that has permanently impacted my overall health. It's also had a profound impact on every aspect of my life, from my ability to work and socialize to things like eating and doing physical activities that I used to enjoy. It's impacted my self-esteem and sense of identity in ways that are very tough to face. And oddly enough, after all

those years of being told the pain was "all in my head" or that I was stressed or depressed or anxious, now that I've been through all of this and I have so much illness and pain in my life day to day, I certainly did become stressed, depressed, and anxious as a result.

I haven't dealt with severe menstrual pain, but I relate to Abby. For me, the mythology around menstruation was more painful than periods themselves. The belief that nature made me a second-class citizen was enough to cause depression, anxiety, and compromised self-esteem. That's a discomfort women all suffer from. We suffer from the emotional pain of believing we're poorly designed. As Roya King, a retired bishop who's worked to combat negative views of menstruation, puts it: "I think women loathe the physical pain because they have the emotional pain with it. A lot of women don't have a grasp on what the body is doing those three to five days out of the month. They don't realize that they're not weakened by it. They don't realize that they are not contaminated from it. They don't realize that they are not despised because of it." When women in one Greek study recounted learning about menstruation, they reported thinking, "Being a woman is dreadful" and "God, I don't want to be a woman."[52] The normalization of menstrual pain makes women feel "physically inferior" and "dislike their own bodies," says Orbuch. When I was told I'd be in pain every month for decades, I felt hated – by nature, by God, by whom, I can't say. It was in fact a millennia-old hatred engraved in history, yet one that was not set in stone.

Chapter 2

Women's Natural Defectiveness and Other Greek Myths

I'm about to travel back in time again to pay a visit to the ancient Greek philosophers. But first, let's make a pitstop at December 2, 2021 – the day my clitoris began failing me. I was thirty-one and excited to receive an invitation from a Bumble match after two years off dating apps: "Want to come over for tea?" Yet when his hand drifted downward later that night, all I could say was, "Gentler, please" (I'm polite in my hookups). No touch seemed gentle enough. So, we transitioned to a cuddle session as I grumbled in my mind about these Bumble dudes and their awkward fingering. But when I touched myself the next day, it hadn't gone away: My clit felt like it was on fire. I couldn't blame the Bumble dudes this time.

The first friend of mine to hear this story said that maybe my clit hurt because I didn't shave. Another said it was normal for the clitoris to be hyper-sensitive. My acupuncturist advised I put castor oil on it and avoid seeing a doctor, as that would start "a whole process." When I finally saw a gynecologist, he recommended pelvic floor physical therapy, since everything "looked fine" from his perspective. Perhaps it was a muscle or nerve issue. Two months later, I got in with a physical therapist, who concluded that things did not, in fact, look fine.

There were signs of a yeast infection, and apparently, you can get a yeast infection in your clitoris. Thankfully, she knew a doctor who confirmed this diagnosis – balanitis – and gave me a topical cream. After five months unable to masturbate comfortably or have sex, I woke up one morning, reached between my legs, and felt what a normal clitoris felt like. It was not "hyper-sensitive." And no, I did not have to shave.

The most painful part once more was not the physical issue but the emotions it brought up: the fear that I wouldn't be able to enjoy this vital body part again. The anger that people weren't taking it seriously. And the knowing deep down that this was happening because my body was seen as unimportant – nonexistent, almost. When I googled "balanitis," I found pages and pages of information about the penis but nothing about the clitoris. "Balanitis is an inflammation of the glans penis," the National Institutes of Health told me. "Balanitis is pain and inflammation (swelling and irritation) of the glans (head) of the penis," the Cleveland Clinic concurred. "Balanitis is soreness and redness in the head of your penis," WebMD echoed.[1] I was trying to be proactive and learn about my body, but all I could see was "penis, penis, penis" all over my screen.

Eyeless Moles and Inverted Genitals

So, yes, the ancient Greeks. Given their limited understanding of science – and women – they developed some colorful concepts of female anatomy. Aristotle speculated that women's bodies were too cold to produce semen, which he considered the source of a child's spirit. Without such spiritual abilities, women simply served as vessels for babies to grow. "The female is, as it were, a mutilated male, and the catamenia [menstrual blood] are semen, only not pure; for there is only one thing they have not in them, the principle of soul," he wrote.[2] While male genitals were "protruding," he observed, "the part under the pubes is hollow or receding" for women. (Yes, that word was "pubes"; it likely refers to the lower abdomen.)[3] Aristotle also stated that "females are weaker and colder in nature" and "we should regard women's nature as suffering from natural defectiveness."[4]

Five centuries later, Galen, the Greek physician who laid modern medicine's foundation, pontificated that women's genitals were like moles' eyes, which don't open or see – "nor do they project but are left there imperfect." The same way moles' eyes were an incomplete version of other animals' eyes, "within mankind, the man is more perfect than the woman," Galen wrote.[5] Aside from that minor point, though, the sexes were the same: "Turn outward the woman's, turn inward, so to speak, and fold double the man's, and you will find the same in both in every respect."[6] This idea endured for centuries: In the 1200s, Italian priest Thomas Aquinas described women as "deficiens et occasionatus," meaning "defective and misbegotten" or, in more generous translations, "unfinished and caused accidentally."[7]

This view of women as lesser men is known by historians as the one-sex model. And while it's easy to feel outrage toward its pioneers, they were on to something. Male and female genitals start off the same in the womb and function similarly in adulthood, complete with erectile tissue, a head covered by a hood or foreskin, and a scrotum or labia made from the same folds.[8] These facts should spawn a sense of equality. Female anatomy *is*, as Aristotle and Galen suggested, like inverted male anatomy. Except it's not inverted. Along with vaginas, females have vulvas and clitorises, which are "protruding." Yet even today, we describe women like incomplete men, calling their entire genitalia the "vagina" – and the intricate, muscular vagina a "hole." While female bodies *are* a lot like male ones (and some bodies defy this binary, which I'll discuss in chapter 4), this idea makes science neglect women under the mistaken belief that studying men tells us all we need to know.

The Clitoris Is Hard to Find ... in Books

For centuries, people assumed women's bodies were, as Aristotle and Galen suggested, empty vessels. As late as the 1500s, European scientists quibbled over whether the clitoris was a normal female feature or a masculine mutation reserved for "hermaphrodites" and lesbians.[9] It took two more centuries for midwives to realize the pelvis pushed the baby out during birth, rather than just laying there as the child journeyed through.[10] Textbooks up through the 1980s and 90s contained details about the penis but no descriptions of the clitoris, with the widely used *Last's Anatomy*'s 1985 edition calling female genitalia a "failure" of male development.[11]

Most disturbingly, certain aspects of female anatomy are still absent from medical education. In 2019, only two popular anatomy textbooks described the clitoral nerves and blood vessels, leaving doctors in the dark about this crucial organ – including surgeons operating on and around it. This is one reason over a thousand botched labiaplasties occur each year, leaving women with diminished sensation and pain. Some received non-consensual clitoral hood reductions due to doctors' ignorance of the clitoral nerves' placement and importance – only to have their pleasurelessness dismissed as normal or a result of not being "in love," as one victim recalled.[12] Because women's genitals are already seen as defective male ones, it doesn't ring nearly enough alarm bells when our genitals *are* damaged or defective.

Which brings me back to my irritated clit. Balanitis in the clitoris works just as it does in the penis: Yeast – or sometimes bacteria – gets under the foreskin or clitoral hood, causing inflammation and pain.[13] Yet the clitoris's health is not taken as seriously as the penis's because the clitoris itself isn't. Nowadays, it's common to hear that the clitoris is "like a small penis" – which, like the Greeks' view of female genitals as inverted male ones, has some truth to it but still defines women by lack. The perception of the clitoris as "small" neglects the internal clitoris, which extends inside the body. The entire clitoris is 3.5–4.3 inches flaccid.[14] The average flaccid penis has been measured at 3.5 inches.[15] Fetuses start off with something more like a clitoris than a penis, so it might be more accurate to describe the penis as a male clitoris.[16] Instead, the clit gets characterized in terms of the penis. The National Library of Medicine defines it as "an erectile structure homologous with the penis," while the penis is "the external reproductive organ of males" – no mention of vulvas.[17] The male is still the default, and women are approached like mutilated men, as Galen put it – or, at best, modified men.

Incomplete Education for Incomplete Men

Sophie Lua grew up in the 1990s in the Netherlands, a country known for excellent sex ed. Yet she remembers learning nothing about female pleasure in school. "They used a condom and a little anatomy chart," she recalls. "It didn't make much of an impact." In the US too, sex ed eschews pleasure, especially female pleasure. Feminist author Peggy Orenstein said it best in her TED talk: "Kids go into their puberty education classes and they learn that boys have erections and ejaculations, and girls have periods and unwanted pregnancy. And they see that internal diagram of a woman's reproductive system – you know, the one that looks kind of like a steer head – and it always grays out between the legs. So we never say 'vulva.' We certainly never say 'clitoris.'"[18] The United Nations International Technical Guidance on Sexuality Education recommends schools teach students about male erections, wet dreams, and ejaculations but says nothing about female erections, arousal, or orgasm.[19]

This invisibilizing of women's anatomy undermines their entitlement to pleasure. After all, it's hard to advocate for attention to body parts you haven't learned the words for. "I used to be really shy talking about it," Sophie says. And when the first four years of her sex life were orgasmless, she didn't think much of it: "I just thought, 'that's how my body is.' I became more aware of it when I started to have a long-term boyfriend, and I thought, 'this is something that's not, I guess, normal, not being able to orgasm.' I'd never really thought that much about it." The vulva's erasure also has huge health ramifications. Stephanie Prendergast, a pelvic floor physical therapist and cofounder of the Pelvic Health and Rehabilitation Center, sees clients with vulvar and clitoral pain conditions that have gone undiagnosed for years. These include a nerve condition called pudendal neuralgia, masses known as keratin pearls that get stuck in the clitoral hood, a vulvar skin condition called lichen sclerosus, and adhesions between the clitoris and clitoral hood.

Many OB/GYNs don't identify these ailments because they don't examine the clitoris. They're focused on the vagina and uterus, reinforcing the view of women's genitals as hollow. "No one's retracting the clitoral hood," Prendergast says. "They're not looking for keratin pearls or infections. These things are not being examined in a woman's routine pap smear." Prendergast says women should retract their clitoral hoods and wash their clitorises daily in the shower to prevent infections or keratin pearls from building up, just as those with uncircumcised penises retract their foreskin. This simple step could prevent many cases of clitoral pain, she says: "Something could be stuck there, like a piece of hair, and they just don't know it's there. Men have to do that in the shower every day; why should we be any different?"

That's the irony: The view of women as incomplete men has prevented us from seeing how we *are* like men, with equivalent body parts requiring equivalent care. And so we don't get that care. In one summer, Prendergast saw eight patients who were misdiagnosed with pudendal neuralgia – the most well-known clitoral pain condition – when they actually had infections, clitoral adhesions, lichen sclerosus, or keratin pearls. She's even seen women undergo unnecessary surgeries for so-called pudendal neuralgia when there was actually an adhesion or infection. "This pathology is affecting more people than is being recognized," she says. "It's misdiagnosed as pudendal neuralgia, or they are being told they have some psychiatric sexual dysfunction – and there is a treatable pathology."

Understudied, Undiagnosed, Untreated

It's not just women's sexuality that has been erased, but women's overall health. Today, only 37% of clinical health trial participants and 24% of drug trial participants are female.[20] Not even animals can escape this bias: Single-sex neuroscience research on male animals is 5.5 times as common as that on females.[21] And this has consequences for humans. Because women themselves are understudied, predominantly female illnesses are poorly understood and go untreated. This includes serious illnesses like fibromyalgia, chronic fatigue syndrome, and chronic Lyme disease – which are still not recognized by many doctors – as well as some shockingly common, everyday issues.[22]

In 2008, America Ramirez came down with a terrible urinary tract infection (UTI). "No pee would come out after trying at least twenty times, but the urgency and burning were so intense that I could not sleep, nor sit or focus on anything else," she recalls. Her doctor diagnosed her with a UTI based on a dipstick test – where you pee in a cup, then a plastic bacteria-detecting stick goes in the urine – and put her on antibiotics. But she recovered only to relapse. After another round of antibiotics, she relapsed yet again. So she saw a urologist, who diagnosed her with an incurable bladder disease called interstitial cystitis (IC). That's when he told her there was no treatment available for this condition. Unwilling to give up, America saw an IC specialist. "She was horrible – made me feel like I was crazy and talked down to me about my symptoms," she says. "From 2008 to 2010, I just suffered. I just dealt with the constant fire in my bladder daily." She finally found a better doctor, but the best she could do was put America on five medications to take four times a day. These suppressed some of her symptoms but did not get rid of them. Even though America's doctors knew this started with a UTI, they overlooked the possible role of bacteria in her pathology. She remembers:

> Having a bladder that feels like someone is pouring acid on it every single day is mentally, emotionally, and physically exhausting. Depression, anxiety, PTSD, agoraphobia, and low self-esteem. Marital issues followed because since I remarried, I would always worry that my husband would tire of my health issues and leave me or cheat on me, since the bladder is affected a lot by sexual activity. I would hurt for days after intercourse, which would make me mentally dread it and of course caused me paranoia about my relationship. I am part of many IC support groups on Facebook. Many of my Facebook IC friends have committed suicide from the pain.

I know this story well. I was diagnosed with this same condition, interstitial cystitis, a decade after America. I can attest to the feeling of acid constantly poured into the bladder. IC, which is twice as common in women, can stem from many issues including pelvic floor muscle dysfunction, infections, food sensitivities, hormonal imbalances, and endometriosis; researchers have called it endometriosis's "evil twin."[23] All these issues can be treated or cured. Yet nearly every medical resource, from the Mayo Clinic to Johns Hopkins Medicine, describes IC as unexplained and incurable.[24] I, like America, was offered nothing but a cocktail of medications to mitigate symptoms. My doctor said the same way some people have sensitive stomachs, others just have sensitive bladders. Another IC patient I interviewed was told by her physician: "This is just like having blue or brown eyes; you were destined to have it."[25] It always seems to be women who "just have" or are "destined to have" bodily problems. I grew depressed as I perused online forums describing IC as permanent, attempting to make peace with the idea that this was how my body was designed. That familiar sense of biological inferiority crept in.

"There's Nothing We Can Do" – Or Is There?

What America and I both had was actually a urinary tract infection – something highly curable. But the standard dipstick tests employed to detect UTIs miss a quarter of infections.[26] Even on more sensitive tests called midstream urine cultures, 20–30% of people with UTI symptoms like bladder pain and frequent urination test negative.[27] New diagnostic methods are revealing that many – likely most – of these patients do indeed have UTIs. PCR tests, for instance, which detect bacterial DNA, have identified infections in patients who tested negative via urine cultures.[28] These infections get missed because patients are harboring a different kind of bacteria than the type tested for, *E. coli*, or the *E. coli* levels are too low for the cultures to pick up.[29] In a 2017 study, 96% of women with UTI symptoms tested positive for *E. coli* on PCR tests, compared to just 68% on midstream urine culture tests. Asymptomatic women tested positive on less than 12% of PCR tests, suggesting the symptoms are indeed from the bacteria. It's just not always detected. "These findings suggest that almost all women with typical urinary complaints and a negative culture still have an infection with *E. coli*," the authors wrote.[30]

Yet many people with UTIs – particularly chronic, low-grade ones – receive the doomful diagnosis of IC, sending them down years-long spirals of misery and body hatred. All because we lack adequate methods for diagnosing UTIs, which at least half of women experience multiple times in their lives.[31] "Given the current science and inability of standard UTI tests to reliably detect chronic UTIs, we find it difficult to accept a diagnosis of interstitial cystitis as a satisfactory outcome for someone experiencing chronic lower urinary tract symptoms," says Andrea Sherwin, spokesperson for Chronic UTI Australia. Could this diagnostic shortcoming exist because UTIs are four times more common in women than men?[32] "Chronic UTI is one of several health conditions predominantly affecting women that are traditionally neglected in medical research and practice," says Sherwin. "We believe gender bias is one reason, although not the only reason, why scientific evidence on UTI diagnosis and treatment has not translated into new, more accurate clinical tests and better treatments."

In a 2023 survey of 410 chronic UTI patients, 96.5% of them female, over 80% struggled to find healthcare providers who could treat their condition. Just as many agreed with the statement: "I have felt that my symptoms have been dismissed or not believed by a healthcare professional."[33] They recounted comments from doctors including: "This just happens to some women," "all women live in pain and [you] need to get used to it," and "sometimes young women get these problems and there's nothing we can do." It's no wonder women's pain is so common it appears normal when we cannot even treat the most basic female maladies. As long as women's bodies are erased from science, medicine, and everyday discourse, their needs will be erased as well. As long as we treat women like inferior men, their lives will indeed be inferior. As long as we see them as cursed, they will be.

Chapter 3

From Stained Sheets to White Houses: The Painful Price of Pleasure

I left out one part of Eve's curse: the part where God says, "Your desire will be for your husband, and he will rule over you." Women were to be under men's control. There's a parallel here, too, with the advent of agrarian societies, which established male control by keeping tabs on women's sexuality. And so virginity became of concern. Deuteronomy, which was written well into agricultural times in the seventh century BC, states that if a man accuses his bride of not being a virgin, her parents should "display the cloth before the elders of the town" as counterevidence. This cloth is presumed to be the blood-stained sheet from their wedding night.[1]

It's debated if this passage is really establishing blood as proof of virginity. Aaron Koller, professor of Near Eastern Studies at Yeshiva University, argues that this law served mainly to warn grooms against making such accusations and give women a defense against them. A bloody sheet could easily be faked, and even back then, people knew the hymen wasn't a map of a woman's sexual history.[2] Still, myriad rituals subsequently emerged under this mistaken belief. In medieval Europe, midwives examined soon-to-be brides' hymens to gauge their purity. The medics of yore also took part in idiosyncratic practices like handing a woman a sieve and seeing if it would hold water, having her cross a lake and checking whether it remained clear, studying her urine, and measuring her neck circumference.[3]

From Adam and Eve to T.I. and Vanessa Carlton

Of all these customs, it's hymen exams that lasted. As recently as 2019, rapper T.I. said he accompanied his eighteen-year-old daughter to the gynecologist for annual hymen checks.[4] A 2018 World Health Organization report revealed virginity tests were taking place in two dozen countries, including places one might not suspect like Canada and the Netherlands.[5] In many parts of the world, from Armenia to Georgia to Polynesia to Australia, some brides' parents still check their sheets for blood to assess their virginity.[6] Most prevalently and powerfully, women across the globe expect first-time sex to involve blood and pain.

I remember when Vanessa Carlton's single "White Houses" came out in 2004. I was thirteen, and a friend told me it was about losing your virginity. When I listened to the lyrics, I learned what this entailed: "a rush of blood and a little bit of pain." Carlton sang to her virginity's recipient that "what I gave is yours to keep."[7] It sounded violating yet somehow romantic: This was a sacrifice for your partner, a sign of love. A couple years later, another friend recounted losing her virginity "to get it over with." At least the pain was now behind her. I wondered why I'd want to have sex. It sounded violent, like something a man took from a woman – along with her innocence. Then in college, I came across an article online saying the hymen didn't need to tear but could stretch. I began questioning the bleak ideas around me. I bought my first vibrator at eighteen, and to my relief, it didn't hurt when

I used it internally. But when I told a couple friends I thought first-time sex would feel good, they suggested I lower my expectations lest they be crushed. "Expect it to hurt," one said. I felt unlucky to be female, just as I did when I learned about periods. I felt foolish for believing life in this vessel could be pleasant.

Around the same time in the aughts, twenty-year-old college student Amanda was becoming sexual with her first boyfriend.[8] She, too, had learned first-time sex was painful – and unfortunately, her experience lived up to that. "It felt horrible; it hurt a lot," she remembers. "I was hopeful that it would get better the second time, and it felt pretty much just as bad – just like being scraped from the inside." She heard other women tell similar stories, so she thought this was normal. She not only resented being a woman but resented men for hurting women so much. She didn't know what she could do about it; her sex ed had been "heavy on the fear factor" but light on practical advice. And her mom's sex talk was limited to "something about how God would be really disappointed in me," she recalls. Was she feeling the wrath of God in her vagina?

Vestiges of the Virgo Intacta

It's easy to think painful sex is natural if we buy into common ideas about female anatomy. If women are not designed for pain, why does the hymen exist? Well, here's some surprising news: It doesn't. Not in the way we think. The hymen is not a seal over the vagina that must break to enable penetration, as the term – from the Greek word for "membrane" – suggests.[9] It's a thin layer of tissue that only partially covers the vaginal opening. In 2009, the Swedish Association for Sexuality Education renamed the hymen the vaginal corona to reflect that it's more like a ring than a membrane.[10] Less than half of women – 34–45% in recent surveys – bleed during their first time, and only 48% of girls who have had intercourse show signs of hymenal tearing. This means most would be classified as "virgins" by onlookers who believe the hymen signals virginity.[11] After examining over 1,000 sexually experienced adolescents' hymens, forensic pediatricians Emma Curtis and Camille San Lazaro reported in the *British Medical Journal* that visible damage is unusual: "In the prepubertal girl, because of the relative size of the structures, penetration occurs through the hymenal tissue and causes tearing; in the adolescent girl and adult woman consensual penetration occurs into the orifice which thus stretches and yields. ... So-called rupture and bleeding of the hymen is not to be routinely expected."[12] In other words, no one has to "pop" anyone's "cherry."

People looking to dispel hymen myths often state that some hymens need not tear during sex because they're already torn from biking, horseback riding, or gymnastics. But one Harvard study found no differences between the hymens of girls who participated in these activities and those who hadn't.[13] To explain why some hymens don't tear during first-time sex, we need not assume they already tore. They don't have to. The hymen becomes more elastic during puberty, allowing it to stretch for penetration – though often it's so small, it doesn't need to.[14] It's almost as if women weren't meant to suffer through sex! The hymen doesn't have many blood vessels, so bleeding is more often due to inadequate arousal, overly rough (unfortunately sometimes non-consensual) intercourse, or medical issues like low estrogen. The "blood on the sheets" believed to stem from hymen tearing may be attributable to vaginal lacerations. And hymens that do tear often heal completely in a matter of days.[15] Someone might have an imperforate hymen, which covers the vaginal opening – or a septate hymen, which stretches vertically over it, partially blocking it – but both are rare and removable through minor surgery.[16]

Scientists have formed fascinating theories about the hymen. Some argue that it evolved to assure women's partners they won't raise another man's child, or that the pain deterred our forebears from sex outside monogamous relationships. Not even our cavewoman ancestors are exempt from today's slut shaming – or the decree that their husbands "rule over" them. Yet as OB/GYN Jen Gunter points out in *The Vagina Bible*, these theories stand on flimsy grounds. Even if a woman's partner is her first and her hymen appears to "prove" so, she could still end up pregnant from someone else further down the line. And the supposed pain of sex certainly doesn't dissuade many modern women from casual hookups or multiple partners. The hymen may instead serve to keep dirt out of the vagina, as it's extra sensitive before puberty, Gunter postulates.[17] It also may protect against bacteria.[18]

Though we know more now than in the Middle Ages, today's doctors offer equally medieval practices in the name of valuing virginity. For hymenoplasties, surgeons construct a hymen using hymenal remains and/or vaginal tissue so women can appear virginal for their wedding nights. Some "revirgination" procedures also involve tightening the vaginal walls under the false belief that sex makes them "loose."[19] And even in recent decades, the old Latin term "virgo intacta" – "untouched virgin" – has been used by lawyers and forensic physicians to evaluate sexual assault accusations.[20] While this phrase has fallen out of favor, hymen exams are still employed in sexual abuse cases, with "normal" findings casting doubt on victims' claims and discouraging them from pressing charges.[21] Yet only 2–4% of child sexual abuse victims show signs of hymenal damage, and hymen size is a poor indicator of past trauma.[22] The virgo intacta is an outdated, misapplied concept, not a medical reality. But even as science shatters myths around it, its cultural vestiges remain intact.

No Cause, or No Knowledge?

The reason we normalize painful sex has less to do with the hymen than what spawned the hymen myth in the first place: the view of women's bodies as made for pain, not pleasure. If you doubt this, look no further than the women whose pain is normalized long after their first time. When Tara Langdale-Schmidt first experienced burning, stabbing sensations during intercourse, she'd had sex before – yet her pain was dismissed all the same. "I would go to my gynecologist," she remembers. "I would tell him 'it's getting worse and worse,' and he literally said – and it's crazy how many people hear this – 'just relax, drink some wine.' I'm like, 'I don't like wine. That makes me feel worse.'" The only alternative he offered was to inject her vulva with lidocaine, a local anesthetic, right before she planned to have sex, which did nothing for her pain – but impeded her pleasure. "He just poked me with a needle like eight to ten times in the most raw spot in my body," she recalls. "You really think I'm gonna go home and have sex? That just doesn't add up."

She started doing her own research and learned about vulvodynia – pain or discomfort in the vulva. Vulvodynia affects 13–16% of women at some point and, like IC and endometriosis, is considered "idiopathic" or without known cause by the medical community.[23] But vulvodynia has many causes; doctors just aren't typically trained to look for them. In 2015, a group of women's health organizations identified seven types of disorders that can cause vulvodynia, including infectious, inflammatory, and hormonal disorders.[24] The infection I had in my clitoris, in fact, was originally diagnosed as "vulvodynia." It's a label frequently slapped on to vulvar pain without further investigation, as if naming a symptom constitutes a diagnosis.

Still, for Tara, it was a step forward to have a word for her condition. She found a new doctor who agreed she had vulvodynia, but even he just suggested antidepressants. "He did not examine me; he didn't touch me," she recalls. "What if I had vulvar or cervical cancer?" Driven online for answers, she connected with other vulvodynia patients and realized many had co-occurring issues like back injuries, connective tissue disorders, gastrointestinal issues, allergies, and chemical sensitivities. Tara herself has been diagnosed with a connective tissue disorder called Ehlers-Danlos syndrome and fibromyalgia, a neurological disorder involving musculoskeletal pain and chronic fatigue. Vulvodynia is two to three times more common in those with fibromyalgia, irritable bowel syndrome, or interstitial cystitis, suggesting some common underlying cause.[25]

Yet with research in its infancy, painful sex masquerades as yet another one of those things women deal with because ... well, because we're women. After tweeting about painful sex, I've received replies like "sex is often painful for women ... [it's] a natural consequence of repeatedly inserting a rigid object into a delicate passageway." But couldn't sex just as easily be described as a powerful muscular organ engulfing a sensitive one?[26] The problem isn't women's bodies but the self-fulfilling view of them as weak and vulnerable – and the conditions we consequently don't treat. Painful sex can also stem from endometriosis, vaginismus (involuntary tightening of the vagina), fibroids, and more.[27] On top of that, one in four women suffers from a pelvic floor disorder – a dysfunction of the muscles surrounding the vagina, anus, and bladder, leading to urinary incontinence, pelvic pain, and/or painful sex.[28] "I don't understand why every woman doesn't know what all the pelvic floor conditions are and how to treat them," Tara says. Maybe it's because pain is still seen as the price women pay for pleasure.

Too Young to Enjoy Sex ... Then Too Old

No, painful sex is not just normalized for newbies – it's also normalized for those deemed past their prime. Due to dropping estrogen levels drying and thinning out the vaginal lining, many women experience painful sex during menopause – and their doctors don't talk about it.[29] Only one in five menopausal women in one Case Western University study were asked about sexual health by their providers. The majority did not bring it up themselves either, most often because they thought their symptoms were a natural part of aging or not bothersome enough to warrant attention.[30] Age, like gender, leads people to dismiss their symptoms as normal and neglect them. In a 2021 survey of 1,000 American women going through menopause, 61% experienced painful sex due to vaginal dryness – but 41% of those women had never used lube or toys, and a quarter were unfamiliar with hormone replacement therapy.[31] Tara, who now runs a tech company geared toward those with vulvodynia, has spoken to countless older women who don't know how to prevent painful sex. "You are fifty, sixty, seventy years old, and still, in your entire life, no one has given you a list of pelvic pain conditions or said 'this is gonna happen after menopause,'" she says. "They're just mind-blown: 'Why didn't people tell me?' Women are left to search for themselves on the internet, and they just suffer in silence." Joan Price, a sex educator focused on aging, echoes:

> We need to educate our medical system about how to diagnose and then alleviate the pain and discomfort that vagina owners often – not always, but often – feel. We need to see all this not as a defect in our bodies but as an opportunity to explore other ways to have wonderfully satisfying sex, arousal, orgasm, and pleasure. We need to celebrate what we've got because our bodies are capable of great sensual and sexual pleasure

lifelong. I think we normalize that getting old means a decrease in pleasure, a decrease in capability.

This point calls for clarification on the difference between normal, natural, and common issues. I have suggested that menstrual pain and pain during sex are common but not normal or natural. Genital discomfort during menopause, however, is both common and sometimes natural but not normal. Aging-related sexual changes frequently occur without an underlying illness, but nobody needs to put up with the discomfort. Oxford Languages defines "normal" as "conforming to a standard; usual, typical, or expected."[32] Given how much it interferes with someone's quality of life, painful sex shouldn't be "expected" at any age, especially with so many options to prevent it. And our "standard" for women's sex lives should be higher, even if certain aspects of aging are natural. Plus, sexual problems aren't always natural even after menopause – and normalizing them can leave health problems undiagnosed. Many conditions behind pelvic pain can afflict someone at any age. Telling older women to "just use more lubricant" can impede the uncovering of pelvic floor dysfunction, yeast infections, and cysts, Joan points out in her book *The Ultimate Guide to Sex After Fifty*.[33] She elaborated in a phone call with me:

> There are many different causes of vaginal pain. You need to have it diagnosed by someone who is a specialist in that area. That means finding an appropriate person who is knowledgeable enough to run the various tests to find out where you are feeling pain: Is it the opening? Is it the inside skin tearing? That's why there are whole specialists in sexual pain, and there are regular doctors who have referral lists to these people: so when someone comes in and says "sex hurts," someone doesn't just say "what do you expect? You're old." Instead, they say, "let's get to the bottom of that."

The Painful Price of Sexual Shame

At all ages, the normalization of painful sex is kept alive by one common factor: the stigma against pleasure. Particularly female pleasure outside marriage and reproduction. It's taboo for a "virgin" to enjoy sex because it brings up fears about how she learned to do so. It shows her sexuality exists outside her partner. It's taboo for an older woman to enjoy sex because her sexuality is separate from motherhood or the male gaze; it's for her. It's taboo for women of any age to love sex because it violates purity ideals. Even if not consciously, perhaps sexual pain is seen as punishment for such violations.

Behind the lack of attention women's pain receives is a fear of women's pleasure. Behind the stigma around female desire is the expectation that her desire be for her husband, who rules over her. In a society that limits women's sexuality to reproduction and marriage, a woman without obstacles to sexual satisfaction is a threat. She represents anxieties over men losing control of women. And so we forgot that sex – for women and everyone – should be a source of joy. The King James Bible references "conception" in Eve's curse – "I will greatly multiply thy sorrow and thy conception" – leading some religious authorities to interpret sexual pain as part of God's will. This may explain why painful sex and vaginismus are particularly common among religious Christians and Jews.[34] Not only can religion-based shame spawn pelvic floor tension and tightness, but the view of pain as divinely orchestrated prevents people from getting help.

During biblical times, sexual restrictions may have served a purpose. Retired bishop Roya King believes the Bible emphasized monogamy to protect women from predatory men. But as long as we live under Eve's curse, our theology and society are incomplete. "The biggest problem we have is that we instituted it as a constant, consistent belief," says King. Whether or not we believe God cursed Eve, it is people who perpetuate her descendants' pain. Not even the Bible says God wanted women's pain to last forever. Not even the Bible says *people* should multiply women's sorrow. Yet through our poor sex education, substandard medical care, and sex-negativity, that's what we've done. Every time we call women cursed, we curse them.

Chapter 4

Men's Bodies Are from Mars, Women's Are from Venus

"**H**as your clitoris always been this large?" Author and activist Hida Viloria is intersex – born with biology that's not strictly male or female. S/he has a uterus and menstruates but never developed secondary sex characteristics like breasts and hips.[1] And the size of he/r clitoris has made he/r the object of questions like this New York City doctor's. The appointment was distressing, as it followed a surgery for a nearly fatal ectopic pregnancy from a rape.[2] Rather than offer support, the doctor scrutinized Hida's body, saying she wanted to "run tests" because he/r clitoris "wasn't normal." Hida recalls: "I could feel her stigmatizing gaze. I felt very insulted and said 'no' and never saw her again."

Intersex people have been recognized throughout the world by many names, including "hermaphrodite" for centuries in Western culture. Today, "intersex" is the most common term for the wide range of people born with sex characteristics that defy standard definitions of male and female, or are a blend of male and female. Up to one in fifty-nine people are born with intersex traits – similar to the number of green-eyed or red-haired people worldwide.[3] Some people are visibly intersex at birth, while others are not until puberty. Others still have chromosomal intersex variations and internal differences that are not physically apparent at all. Hida saw a different doctor a decade later to find out which intersex variation s/he had, recalling:

> She kept asking me which I felt more like, a man or a woman. This was during a time period where I looked very androgynous. I explained that that wasn't the issue; I just wanted medical tests ... but she kept asking. When I told her I felt like both, she wasn't satisfied and said that "if I had to choose," which one would I choose, man or woman? It was very frustrating and shocking to me that a medical doctor felt the need to try to psychologically figure me out and squeeze me into the male/female binary that I was literally born outside of just to treat me. But this is very typical of how the medical establishment treats intersex people.

From One Sex to Two

To understand how women came to be physically ranked below men, we need to look at how bodies were split into opposing "male" and "female" categories in the first place. As the late 1600s rang in the Age of Enlightenment, religion held less weight in European thinking. Instead, science served to enforce gender norms. In light of medical discoveries of sex differences, the one-sex model gave way to what historians call the two-sex model. Under this philosophy, women weren't inverted or inferior men; they were men's polar opposite – but still inferior. This idea gained traction in the ensuing two centuries as political forces confined women to the home. "A perfect woman and a perfect man ought not to resemble each other ... one ought to be active and strong, the other passive and weak," professed Swiss philosopher Jean-Jacques

Rousseau in 1762.[4] "Woman is a pair of ovaries with a human being attached, whereas man is a human being furnished with a pair of testes," wrote nineteenth-century German doctor Rudolf Virchow.[5] An 1895 issue of the French magazine *La Plume* declared women "the weaker sex" with "no business competing in public life," as "a woman exists only through her ovaries."[6]

Femaleness and maleness became defining characteristics no one could escape. In 1803's *Natural History of Women*, French physician Jacques-Louis Moreau declared that "all the points of [a woman's] being reveal her sex and present a series of oppositions and contrasts to all the corresponding parts of men." A woman is a woman "in all manners of existence, in her moral affections as in her physical system, in her joys as well as her suffering," he proclaimed.[7] Another French physician, Jean-Louis Brachet, echoed in 1847 that "all parts of [a woman's] body present the same differences: All express woman; the brow, the nose, the eyes, the mouth, the ears, the chin, the cheeks. If we shift our view to the inside, and with the help of the scalpel, lay bare the organs, the tissues, the fibers, we encounter everywhere ... the same difference."[8]

Today, we express this credo by professing that men and women are from different planets. In the popular self-help book *Men Are from Mars, Women Are from Venus*, which sold 6.6 million copies in the 1990s, relationship counselor John Gray writes that "brain and hormonal differences" between men and women have created opposing social needs, communication styles, and more – and while perhaps one in ten women act like "Martians," this is frequently due to high testosterone.[9] While allowing some flexibility, this leaves the two-sex system in place, acknowledging "masculine" women yet painting them as less female. While hormones impact behavior, testosterone and estrogen play diverse roles, many of them unaligned with what we consider "masculine" and "feminine." Estrogen is a driver of libido in women, and testosterone promotes bonding and helpfulness in men.[10] Our hormones, like us, are similar. Yet the centuries-old belief that men and women are biologically alien continues to impede empathy on Earth. Here, it seems there's room for Venusians and Martians, but few in between.

"All Based in a Colonial Mindset"

Kuya'karanuta'ni (or Kuya) Gonzalez came down with long Covid in 2021. The ensuing appointments were frustrating due to doctors' poor understanding not just of the condition but of gender. The forms all had two options to check – "male" or "female" – which neglected Kuya's gender and cultural background. Kuya, who is of Afro-Borikua Taíno ancestry and lives in Arizona, identifies as two-spirit – a term for Indigenous people with elements of both male and female gender.[11] Since Kuya's birth sex was female, they checked "female" on the forms, knowing doctors' visits weren't conducive to discussions of identity. It nevertheless felt alienating when staff used "she" and "her" to refer to Kuya, who prefers "they/them" pronouns. "As an Indigenous person, I know that this is all based in a colonial mindset," they explain. "I know that my gender has always been in existence and will always be in existence, and it's very unfortunate when people don't acknowledge that." The misgendering and condescension for being a gender-nonconforming person of color "adds to the sense of unsafety and just not wanting to engage at all ... and feeling very unseen," Kuya shares.

While biological sex differences exist in nature, interpretations of these differences are cultural. And racial oppression has solidified the binary Western gender system. In the Americas, colonizers imposed European gender norms on Indigenous tribes, killing many two-spirit people. Jacques Marquette, a French Jesuit missionary, wrote in 1674 of Indigenous males who "take on women's clothing" and "lower themselves by doing everything that women do."[12] This notion of femininity as "lower" shows how intertwined gender policing is with male supremacy. Though this began before the two-sex model's ascent, there already was a two-gender system based largely on religious roles.[13] Enlightenment-age science cemented these gender roles in biology, presenting them as immutable truths – and depicting those who defied them as unnatural, even as these same roles erased natural human variance.

The Invisibility of Body Diversity

The two-sex model placed those outside the gender and sex binaries under close medical scrutiny. In 1779, English anatomist Thomas Brand set the stage for modern intersex surgeries by altering a seven-year-old's genitalia to fit standards of male anatomy, including larger size and the ability to pee upright "like any other boy." His case study advocated the two-sex model, stating that his patient was male all along and no one was really a hermaphrodite – that era's term for intersex people. "The term 'hermaphrodite' is properly understood as an animal that has both the male and female organs equally and perfectly formed," he wrote. "But ... there is no reason to believe that such a case ever had existence in the human subject."[14]

In reality, there are over thirty genetic and developmental variations of intersex traits in humans.[15] But Brand's legacy has lasted. By the mid twentieth century, forced surgeries on intersex infants and children were routine in the UK and US thanks to later clinicians like psychologist John Money.[16] Today, the intersex community is still campaigning to end non-consensual, unnecessary, and dangerous surgeries to make children appear "normal," including clitoral reductions and penile alterations to enable urination while standing.[17]

Although intersex traits are innate, medicine stigmatizes them. Doctors perpetuate the surgical removal and "correction" of sex variations by calling them "disorders of sex development," Hida explains:

> Medicine fails intersex people because, rather than accepting us as equal human beings, it positions being intersex as a birth defect that should be removed or "corrected" – as infants and minors no less. This assumption is why the medical establishment as a whole has ignored hundreds of reports from intersex adults that they were harmed by these surgeries – and why these surgeries persist.

How Many Sexes ... and Genders?

Today, there remains debate over how many sexes exist, with some arguing that since everyone produces either sperm or eggs, there are two.[18] Others point to the diversity of genitalia (male, female, or intersex), gonads (testes, ovaries, or ovotestes), chromosomes (XX, XY, or intersex variations like XO and XXY), and hormones in the human population.[19] Alongside this debate over sex, which refers to biology, scientists and politicians alike are concerned with how many genders – social identities – are legitimate. These questions are intertwined, as gender norms influence sex classifications; they're why many can only conceive of "male" and "female." And biology in turn may influence gender: Some research suggests hormonal factors contribute to gender identity.[20] Gender diversity, like sex diversity, is a natural part of the human species, with hundreds of cultures recognizing more than two genders.[21] But this group is similarly fighting for the right to be respected rather than pathologized. It wasn't until 2013 that the Diagnostic and Statistical Manual removed "gender identity disorder" as a diagnosis for therapists to give clients simply for being transgender.[22] It's not just women but also trans, non-binary, two-spirit, and intersex people – a group I'll describe with the umbrella term "sex and gender-diverse people" – whom medicine's confines deem defective.

So, it's no wonder that sex and gender-diverse people's pain gets normalized along with women's. Ed, a non-binary trans man in the UK, faced "unpredictable waves of agonizing pain" due to ovarian cysts and polycystic ovary syndrome. His menstrual cramps had "always been bad before; sometimes I couldn't walk," he recalls. "A couple times in my early twenties, I passed out on the bathroom floor. But these were worse and left me screaming. This devastated my social and work life, and I spent most of my time at home." His doctor trivialized these symptoms with comments like "life is a mysterious basket of pains." Ed wanted to treat them by getting a hysterectomy, or uterus removal, but could not until a gender identity clinic testified it was in his "psychiatric best interests." It took months to finally get a letter, then he had to explain trans identity to an administrator who said, "We don't do this procedure on men."

Iain Birchall, another UK trans man, similarly struggled to get a Depo-Provera shot for period pain. The "contraceptive" section of his records was grayed out since he identified as male. "This also means that there's no flag to send me any pap smear test reminders," he says. When he calls to book appointments, staff ask if it's for his "wife" or say, "You do know that's for women, right?" he recounts. "So essentially, I have no privacy because I have to out myself at first point of contact. You'd think they'd have the common sense to realize that transitioning doesn't wave a magic wand, and you still need access to medical care for some aspects of your birth sex. My thinking is they shouldn't restrict it in the first place; there's no need to." Gendered beauty standards also enter medical settings: Another doctor told Iain he knew a surgeon who "could have done better" when observing scars from his chest surgery. "It's exhausting being judged on how well you pass and perform by medical professionals when it's just none of their bloody business," he says. On the flip side, social worker Shanéa P. Thomas has seen trans clients' complaints brushed off by doctors because they conformed to beauty ideals. When one trans woman she worked with expressed concern about her hormone levels, her physician said everything must be fine because she looked "beautiful."

At best, many providers simply don't know how to treat bodies outside the two-sex model's limits. In a 2022 *Washington Post* survey, half of trans people said their doctors knew little to nothing about transgender healthcare.[23] In the 2015 US Transgender Survey, a third of trans people who'd recently seen healthcare practitioners reported negative experiences such as harassment, being refused service, and needing to educate their providers.[24] "It's very difficult to find a doctor who knows anything about transgender health," says Rachel, a trans woman in Los Angeles. "I went to a specialist a few years ago who was going to give me a refill on my hormones, so I told him what I was taking. He had to go online and look up what he was supposed to prescribe. There was no way for me to find a transgender-informed physician. I had to call doctors' offices one at a time, and the person who answers does not usually know what you're talking about."

The Myth of Male and Female Health Conditions

The division of medicine into "male" and "female" conditions affects more than just sex and gender-diverse people. It affects anyone with complaints or needs not stereotypically associated with their gender or sex. Shanéa, for instance, identifies as non-binary and uses both she/her and he/him pronouns – but that's not the primary reason she's had trouble getting prescriptions for PrEP, a medication that prevents HIV.

The main reason is simply that his birth sex was female, and people see HIV as a gay men's issue. "I had to almost beg my doctors to get the PrEP, and that's not the same struggle for my gay male friends," Shanéa says. "If I continue to partner with the people I want to partner with, to be able to protect myself and other people, this is something I need for myself. But with doctors' offices and appointments, I'm questioned 'why, why, why?'" It's another way the two-sex model fails us: by seeing certain health issues as gendered when they aren't. In reality, most people living with HIV worldwide are female.[25] Shanéa's experience also illustrates how racism reinforces the medical gender binary: HIV is more common among African American women than White women, so it's overlooked by a system that prioritizes White patients' concerns.[26]

The gendering of bodies also fuels the research gap between "male" and "female" health issues. Some conditions differ in commonality by sex, but few affect only one. Fibromyalgia and interstitial cystitis, for instance, are under-studied in part because they're perceived as female illnesses – but they do affect males more than is acknowledged. And many of these men lack solutions because they have "women's" conditions that are poorly understood and therefore hard to treat. Or, they're assumed to have something else entirely; men with IC are often misdiagnosed with prostatitis.[27] Even endometriosis can occur in males.[28] On the flip side, heart attacks are more common in men, leading them to be overlooked in women. Yet women are more likely to die from heart attacks due to inadequate treatment stemming from the assumption that they don't get them. In addition, heart attack symptoms that are more common in women are less widely recognized.[29] This demonstrates how the one-sex and two-sex models both fall short. The two-sex model leads us to acknowledge certain conditions in only one gender, and the one-sex model leads us to assume they'll look the same in all genders. We need a more nuanced paradigm to understand that most health conditions affect people of all sexes and genders but manifest differently.

Toward a Multi-Sex Model

The one-sex and two-sex models both define women as lacking what men have, whether by having smaller amounts of the same things or having something opposite and inferior. And both erase sex and gender diversity. Perhaps the way out of this system is a multi-sex, multi-gender model like the one Indigenous communities advocate. "The first step is really getting out of that colonial mindset," says Kuya. "Western medicine is based on colonization, so that's the real problem. Before colonization, most Indigenous people recognized more than two genders. Some recognized five genders. Some recognized even more because there are so many nuances to gender. And they acknowledged that two-spirit people are actually sacred because they're able to hold these various genders and identities."

Thinking of gender and sex like multidimensional spectrums also helps us care for men and women, since "male" and "female" traits are not mutually exclusive. As I mentioned in my discussion of balanitis, failing to acknowledge male and female genitals' commonalities can lead to misdiagnoses. And denying similarities between bodies cements social assumptions along with medical ones. Magazines are full of articles framing neuroscience findings as proof men are from Mars while women are from Venus. Yet while there are slight neurological differences between the average man and woman, most people's brains are "mosaic," meaning some regions are more male-typical and others are more female-typical.[30] Denying this perpetuates biases.

Acknowledging diversity, on the other hand, undermines hierarchy. It's difficult to place one sex or gender above others if we see how they're not actually so different. Not in the limited way the one-sex model sees it, but in an expansive way that recognizes bodies from all over the galaxy. Male supremacy looks silly when we see that males have many "female" traits, and vice versa. That's not how the Western, White-dominated medical model currently works, and that has far-ranging implications for our lives beyond our healthcare. As long as we view gender as a biological binary, we'll uphold ideas that place Adam's body above Eve's – and the many bodies in between.

Chapter 5

How the Female Orgasm Became Elusive

Kaytlin Bailey grew up in 1990s North Carolina with a feminist mother who aimed to arm her with information about her body. During her teen years, her mom taught her that "men are so easy and simple and women are so complicated," she recalls. "Female bodies were supposed to be these mystical, magical, incomprehensible things. It wasn't explained to me that people are different – different men, women, and trans people achieve pleasure differently and you just have to figure that out. It was sold to me as this complicated thing." Meanwhile, Kaytlin's aunt described sex as something men took from women, and women's duty was to "get it over with" or "finish the job."

During middle school, Kaytlin and her friends would talk for hours about how to make sex hotter for men, despite how simple they supposedly were. She learned how penises worked from magazines and porn but heard little about vulvas, which compounded their mystique. She first masturbated to orgasm in high school, but her experiences with partnered sex were different. By the time she started having sex at seventeen, she'd internalized that the goal was to please men. So, impressing partners was her focus. Her own orgasms were absent. Later on, while working as an escort, Kaytlin observed that men varied widely, and it took effort to learn how to please them. But because of what she'd learned from her family and culture, she still felt like the complicated one. "Orgasm was sold to me as a mystical experience that was bestowed upon you by a magical power," she says. "A man that could make you come was either a sorcerer or 'the one.'"

Margaret Carmel began her sex life unplagued by such doubts. In high school, she enjoyed her first sexual experiences. Then, during her senior year, a psychiatrist put her on Zoloft to alleviate depression and anxiety, telling her the only side effects to look out for were nausea and drowsiness. Over the next few months, her sexual pleasure ebbed away a bit at a time until she barely felt any. Because of what she'd heard about the "elusive female orgasm," she figured this was part of maturing into womanhood. "I heard that women have difficulty orgasming from reading women's magazines like *Cosmo*," she reflects. "Orgasms for women weren't something that anyone I knew talked about in the casual and accessible way society talks about male orgasms. It felt like having an orgasm as a woman was a pleasure set aside for the select few. In order to have one, you had to be special and have a skilled partner." When she started dating her first boyfriend in college, she realized even a serious relationship wasn't enough. Despite his attempts to please her, she never got aroused or wet, so they didn't end up having intercourse. She felt so little pleasure, she began avoiding intimacy, telling herself perhaps she still lacked the great love required for female orgasm.

During my first eight sexually active years, orgasms seemed elusive to me too. Similar to Margaret, I was put on Prozac – which works like Zoloft – during my senior year of high school without being warned of sexual side effects. Who would expect a single seventeen-year-old girl to care about orgasms? But I did. When I began hooking up in college, I was disappointed not to orgasm with partners. I did alone, but it required lots of time and/or toys, which had not been the case pre-Prozac. After being too embarrassed to bring this up for months, I finally learned from my psychiatrist that it likely related to my meds. But for years, the issue didn't seem important enough to consider stopping them. When I mentioned it to my college nurse, she just told me "lots of women" had that issue and suggested a vibrator. Few partners asked whether or how I might climax. Other women advised me to "just enjoy the journey," and I would. Yet I was quick to accept this suggestion only because the destination seemed unattainable. After all, in the movies and TV shows I'd grown up with, women's climaxes were scarce commodities – from Meg Ryan's head-turning fake orgasm in *When Harry Met Sally* to Charlotte and Carrie's stunned faces when *Sex and the City*'s Samantha says she always comes, to Jerry Seinfeld's joke that "the female orgasm is kind of like the bat cave: Very few people know where it is, and if you're lucky enough to see it, you probably don't know how you got there."[1]

Anti-Feminist Backlash and the Demotion of Female Sexuality

It wasn't always like this. The prevalent beliefs about female orgasm 400 years ago make ours look outdated. In early modern Europe, women's orgasms were deemed essential, thanks to Galen and Hippocrates' theory that they emitted a seed needed for conception.[2] This was an unexpected benefit of the one-sex model: Female orgasms were seen the same way as male ones. They were not considered less attainable, and information on how to attain them was available. Marriage guidebooks taught men to caress their partners' external genitalia. Without the clitoris, "the fair sex neither desire nuptial embraces, nor have pleasure in them, nor conceive by them," reads a 1684 English sex manual describing clitoral anatomy and erections.[3] In the 1740s, when Habsburg Empire ruler Maria Theresa was struggling to conceive, her physician recommended "the vulva of Her Most Holy Majesty should be titillated before intercourse."[4]

Nor were women thought to value sexual pleasure less than men. Pre-Enlightenment European thinkers deemed women *more* libidinous due to Aristotle's equation of men with the spirit and women with the flesh, along with religious views of Eve's descendants as hungry and sin-prone. Medieval Latin priest Jerome wrote in the 400s that "women's love in general is accused of ever being insatiable; put it out, it bursts into flame; give it plenty, it is again in need."[5] A millennium later, the 1486 German witch-hunting guide *Malleus Maleficarum* read that, obviously, witches were mostly women since "all witchcraft comes from carnal lust, which in women is insatiable."[6] The narrative took a turn when word got out that women could conceive without coming. Historian Thomas Laqueur writes in *Making Sex: Body and Gender from the Greeks to Freud* that "the presence or absence of orgasm became a biological signpost of sexual difference" between men and women in the late 1700s.[7] "Medical writings – popular and learned – claimed that women were less given to desiring sexual pleasure and that in any case, it was irrelevant to their reproductive lives," Laqueur elaborated in an email to me. But as usual, there was more to the story than medicine. And it has more to do with my story, Kaytlin's, and Margaret's than you might assume.

Around the time the myth of the elusive female orgasm emerged, multiple European countries were experiencing backlash against gender equality, igniting enthusiasm for sex roles. As the French Revolution spawned a women's movement, anxieties around female power fueled the two-sex model's view of women as weaker. Men entering the bourgeois public sphere dug up physical "evidence" that women shouldn't join them. Louis-Marie Prudhomme, publisher of the *Revolutions of Paris* paper, responded to news of a female political club:

"In the name of nature from which one must never stray, in the name of good domestic morality, of which women's clubs are the scourge ... we implore the good citizenesses of Lyons to stay home and to look after their households." He deemed this the best choice according to "reason and J.J. Rousseau," the Swiss philosopher who believed biology gave men and women different jobs.[8] Such ideas painted the genders as bodily opposites and sexual opposites: Part of women's "natural" role as housewives in eighteenth-century France was "pudeur," or chastity.[9]

Meanwhile, a new feminine ideal in Great Britain also declared women purer and better suited to home life than men. As historian Nancy F. Cott writes in "Passionlessness: An Interpretation of Victorian Sexual Ideology," eighteenth-century British writers "portrayed sexual promiscuity as one of those aristocratic excesses that threatened middle-class virtue and domestic security." Since women were responsible for upholding their households and raising the next generation, they were expected to refrain from sensual pursuits; God forbid they abandon their husbands or corrupt their children. Purity ideals also spread via etiquette guides encouraging female demureness and deference to men's "pleasure and service," Cott writes.[10] Scottish physician John Gregory's 1761 *A Father's Legacy to His Daughters* states that women are "designed to ... polish [men's] manners," as their "superior delicacy" and "modesty" keep them "from any temptation to those vices to which we are most subjected."[11] In England and the colonial US, Evangelical Christianity reinforced propriety for women – particularly White women, whose chastity was established in contrast to allegedly animalistic Indigenous women.[12] And so the belief in women's out-of-control passions receded behind a view of lust as unladylike. British urologist William Acton went as far as to write in 1857 that "the majority of women (happily for them) are not very much troubled with sexual feelings of any kind."[13]

Feminine Sexual Anesthesia: A Century-Old Spell

As women's sexuality became an inconvenience to the social order, science went into denial about the clit. The clitoris in 1901's *Gray's Anatomy* had disappeared in time for the 1948 edition.[14] Some early twentieth-century thinkers outright denied women's ability to feel pleasure outside intercourse within marriage. Dutch gynecologist Theodoor Hendrik van de Velde's 1926 *Ideal Marriage*, the best-known marriage guidebook of its time, claimed women possessed a "less rapid and facile excitability" and could only overcome their "feminine sexual anesthesia" through an "erotic education" from their husbands. He elaborated: "The newly married woman is, as a rule, more or less completely 'cold' or indifferent to and in sexual intercourse."[15] Women required men's help to unlock their pleasure – and only if these men were their husbands. They were far from autonomously orgasmic.

This idea sounds eerily similar to the myths Kaytlin's family taught her: the myth of "the one" needed to awaken a woman's sensuality. The myth of women's reticent pleasure. Maybe that's because modern sex guides – even those geared toward empowerment – reflect similar sentiments. "Guys are so simple. Stroke their penises and they have orgasms. ... A woman's arousal is typically slower and gentler, requiring greater emotional buy-in," *Men's Health* editors Laurence Stains and Stefan Bechtel write in 1996's *Sex: A Man's Guide*.[16] "The female orgasm is a more complicated affair and often takes much longer to achieve," echoes sex therapist Ian Kerner's 2004 bestseller *She Comes First: The Thinking Man's Guide to Pleasuring a Woman*.[17] In 2007's *I Love Female Orgasm*, sex educators Dorian Solot and Marshall Miller describe "bringing a woman to orgasm" as "a slow and challenging process."[18] Even the feminist site *Jezebel* responded to a sad study on women's lack of orgasms in hookups: "Are you sure you want an orgasm

EVERY time? ... Look, orgasms are weird. ... For women, they *are* often more elusive."[19] WebMD offers an article on women "in search of the elusive orgasm," and CNN an investigation into "the purpose of the ever-elusive female orgasm."[20] It seems the consensus is clear, then: Women's orgasms elude everyone.

This was why it didn't seem strange when my first partnered sexual encounters were orgasmless. The message around me was that it was nearly impossible for a human female to reach climax. My freshman year of college, two sex educators staged a comedic performance, complete with a song claiming that "women take forty-five minutes to orgasm." Two years later, when I apologized to my first boyfriend for not climaxing during oral sex, he said, "I know it's harder for girls," then stopped trying. I figured the elusive orgasm was just another way being female was not very fun.

Female Pleasurelessness: Statistics or Society?

There is data demonstrating that women orgasm less often than men. A 2010 Indiana University study of 4,000 Americans found that 91% of men but only 64% of women climaxed during their last encounter.[21] A similar "orgasm gap" has been documented in Canada, Australia, Finland, Russia, and Thailand, uniting women worldwide through shared sexual frustration.[22] There are many theories painting this gap as natural, from the scientific to the spiritual. On the biological end, neuroscientist Louann Brizendine claims in *The Female Brain* that women have a harder time orgasming than men – so much so that they take "three to ten times longer" – because if they orgasm *after* their partners, their vaginal contractions suck in sperm, promoting pregnancy.[23] For this theory to make sense, it would have had to be the norm throughout our evolution that women continued receiving pleasure after their partners' climaxes – unfortunately a flimsy premise. It's also unclear whether women's orgasms assist with impregnation, with some research showing no link between orgasm rates and fertility.[24] Other findings suggest female orgasm could facilitate sperm transport and retention by stimulating a series of uterine contractions called peristalsis. However, peristalsis lasts for minutes, so the woman's orgasm need not follow her partner's for it to have this effect.[25]

On the spiritual side of things, empowerment guru Mama Gena claims women's orgasms require more effort because the vulva knows "she is the most interesting, fascinating, and wonderful thing there is" and "there's no better way for you and your partner to spend your time than pleasing her." Her book *Pussy* professes that "the elusive nature of female orgasm is an opportunity, not a problem. She takes her time because there is no rush."[26] While poetic, this is not based on fact. In 1953's *Sexual Behavior in the Human Female*, sex research pioneer Alfred Kinsey documented that his female subjects orgasmed in slightly under four minutes on average through masturbation – "not appreciably slower than the male." Forty-five percent took one to three minutes, and 12% took over ten. "Certain it is that many males reach orgasm before their wives do in their marital coitus, and many females experience orgasm in only a portion of their coitus," he wrote. "These facts seem to substantiate the general opinion that the female is slower than the male, but our analyses now make it appear that this opinion is based on a misinterpretation of the facts. ... It is true that the average female responds more slowly than the average male in coitus, but this seems to be due to the ineffectiveness of the usual coital techniques."[27] More recently, in 2018, a 3,000-woman survey by Indiana University researcher Devon Hensel and the site OMGYES found the median time frame women took to orgasm alone was five minutes.[28]

Sex therapists and educators routinely publish the statistic that women take twenty minutes to orgasm. Most cite one another without an original source. Some cite textbooks like *Psychology Applied to Modern Life*, which claims sex researchers Masters and Johnson found that women orgasm in ten to twenty minutes during sex. We might attribute this to the "ineffectiveness of the usual coital techniques," as Kinsey put it – were the statistic real. After finding it nowhere in Masters and Johnson's work, I contacted the textbook's co-author Elizabeth Yost Hammer, who said: "My guess – only a guess – is that those original statements were taken from another human sexuality text, who got them from who knows where, and sometime over the first eight editions, the citation was misattributed."[29] The myth of female pleasurelessness leads baseless figures to be passed off as science, remaining unquestioned for years as gender norms seep into classrooms, books, and newsfeeds unannounced.

What is it, then, that makes women orgasm less reliably than men? Some say a woman's sexual response is uniquely dependent on emotions. "Because of the delicate psychological and physiological interconnection, female orgasm has been elusive to confused male lovers," Brizendine writes in a *Female Brain* passage reminiscent of *Ideal Marriage*. "The neurochemical stars need to align. Most important, she has to trust who she's with."[30] Yet the common belief that women must "shut off their minds" to orgasm is questionable. A 2017 Rutgers brain imaging study found "no evidence of deactivation of brain regions leading up to or during orgasm" whether women were alone or with partners.[31] Anxiety and trauma can impede climax for anyone, but perhaps it's not that women *need* more emotional safety than men. If anything, it's that they *have* less thanks to the constant threat of sexual violation.[32]

Contrary to the theories rendering women's orgasms mysterious puzzles, the reason they appear elusive may be simple. When women receive oral and manual stimulation, 90% or more orgasm.[33] And during masturbation, 95% orgasm easily.[34] That's because, unlike intercourse, these activities provide clitoral stimulation. Only one in four women orgasms every time they have penetrative intercourse.[35] This would also explain why the orgasm gap is specific to heterosexual encounters. A 2017 study of 53,000 Americans found that 65% of straight women, compared to 95% of straight men, orgasmed in all or most of the past month's encounters – but the gap between gay men and lesbians was just 89% vs. 86%. "It is quite possible that lesbian women are less likely than heterosexual men to believe that orgasms are elicited primarily by vaginal sex," the authors wrote. "Lesbian women may be more likely to hold sexual script norms regarding equity in orgasm occurrence, including a 'turn-taking culture' where lesbian women ... take turns receiving pleasure until each is satiated."[36]

Why Women's Orgasms Really Seem Elusive

The "elusive female orgasm" is a self-fulfilling prophecy. We have yet to shake the eighteenth-century idea that women are less desiring and capable of orgasms – and don't need them since they're inessential for conception. And because of that, female orgasms aren't valued enough for women to attain them. The clitoris is excluded from our definition of "sex": "sexual activity, including specifically sexual intercourse," Google tells us. "Sexual intercourse" is in turn defined as "sexual contact between individuals involving penetration, especially the insertion of a man's erect penis into a woman's vagina."[37]

Cultural conventions around sex also reflect the myth of female passionlessness. US and Canadian studies have found men receive oral sex far more than women – a dynamic fueled by a "narrative of women's orgasms as work and men's orgasms as natural," one McMaster University study reads.[38] It may indeed feel "unnatural" to stimulate the clit if you can't find it: Though it may finally appear in textbooks, only 56% of American college men could locate it on a diagram as recently as 2010.[39] When women's partners do provide oral or manual sex, it's often not continued to completion but treated as "foreplay" – or "sexual activity that precedes intercourse," to consult Google again.[40] As if the clit merits no attention for its own sake. In 1976's *The Hite Report*, German sex researcher Shere Hite identified a cohort of frustrated women whose partners provided just enough clitoral stimulation to get them excited. "The sequence of 'foreplay,' 'penetration,' and 'intercourse' (defined as thrusting), followed by male orgasm as the climax and end of the sequence, gives very little chance for female orgasm, is almost always under the control of the man, frequently teases the woman inhumanely, and in short, has institutionalized out any expression of women's sexual feelings except for those that support male sexual needs," she concluded.[41]

Hite's subjects debunked the Enlightenment-era – but unenlightened – view of women as lacking desire, airing complaints like "I'm on edge all the time and feel sluggish and congested [if I don't orgasm]." Many women stopped seeking orgasms because they felt like a lost cause, not because they didn't want them. "Supposedly women are less interested in sex and orgasms than men, and more interested in 'feelings,' less apt to initiate sex, and generally have to be 'talked into it,'" Hite wrote. "But the reason for this, when it is true, is obvious: Women often don't expect to, can't be sure to, have orgasms."[42] Due not to their biology but to its neglect.

Evening the (Already Even) Playing Field

Since we've called women's orgasms "elusive" so many times it feels like fact, the orgasm gap's proposed solutions do little to challenge this script. Many instead perpetuate the myth that this gap is innate. Closing the orgasm gap is now a business, with sex toy and lube brands claiming to help women overcome their passionlessness with statistics like "women typically take up to three times longer than men to climax" and testimonials like "that often elusive orgasm was suddenly not so hard to achieve."[43]

Toys may be harmless, but the assumption that women's bodies disadvantage them has spawned riskier solutions. Physicians now offer a variety of procedures to rectify women's orgasmic difficulties. In 2002, gynecologist David Matlock invented an injection called the G-shot, which dozens of physicians around the world offer for around $1,500. It allegedly plumps the G-spot with the filler hyaluronan to increase women's sensitivity.[44] In a 2018 paper, surgeon Adam Ostrzenski detailed another procedure called "G-spotplasty," which he performed on three women by removing tissue where he believed the G-spot was – I say "believed" because it's not visible so would be hard to locate – then stitching it back up to tighten it.[45] Another technique called vaginal fat grafting involves injecting fat cells from body parts like the hips and thighs into the vaginal lining, purportedly tightening the vagina and moving the G-spot outward in case patients' orgasms were hiding in there.[46] I'm sorry to say that's not all: A machine called the Orgasmatron promised to assuage women's orgasmic woes by surgically inserting electrodes into their spines. "Not only am I not normal, I am diseased," a woman laments before trialing this device in the 2009 documentary *Orgasm Inc.* After it sadly does nothing but make her leg twitch, she says she'll just have to embrace sex acts beyond intercourse – she'd climaxed clitorally all along.[47]

But wait, there's more! Hundreds of doctors worldwide administer an injection called the O shot, which purportedly facilitates arousal, lubrication, and orgasm. Blood from the arm is spun in a centrifuge to isolate the platelet-rich plasma (PRP), the genitals are numbed with lidocaine, then the PRP is injected into the clitoris, along with a place in the vagina O shot inventor Charles Runels calls the "O spot" (not a medically recognized body part, if you haven't guessed).[48] "I've found a lot of women don't orgasm, or have the inability to orgasm during intercourse," former *Real Housewives of New York City* star Cindy Barshop, whose "vagina spa" VSPOT offers the O shot, told a local magazine. "It's something that's very simple and can be fixed and we should be doing it."[49] In 2016, I received an email from VSPOT's PR rep describing several procedures "dedicated to empowering women through their ladybits," including the O shot – and inviting me to try it. At that time, having never orgasmed from anyone's touch but my own, I felt desperate to cultivate a sex life free from dysfunction. So, after Barshop reassured me I would "not feel a thing," I found myself in the VSPOT OB/GYN's office. "If this doesn't work, you should consider a clitoral hood reduction," she said. "That way, your partners won't have to pull the hood back. Your clitoral hood covers your clitoris, so that could be your problem." I lay there ashamed as she administered the shot, wondering if my anatomy had hindered my pleasure – even though I'd orgasmed easily by touching my clitoral hood. I never had to "pull it back." Nor was it hard to touch the glans directly, though that felt *too* intense.[50] I had no lack of sensitivity. Spoiler alert: The shot did nothing.

While neither Kaytlin nor Margaret were aware they could be "fixed" this way, both say they felt "broken." Margaret recalls: "Every time my body did not cooperate with what my brain wanted to do, I always lay there feeling broken and down." This sense of brokenness doesn't just belong to individuals; it's layered on top of a belief that women are broken for being women. No matter what we do to rectify our own anatomy, these alterations won't disrupt the perception of a flawed female core. One woman wrote to sex educator Betty Dodson in 2009: "Much of the time I hate being a female because it is IMPOSSIBLE for me to orgasm through sex ...

why did God make it so difficult for women to orgasm and so easy for men?"[51] One of Hite's subjects said not orgasming "feels like someone is trying to kill me, like God hates me by not letting me be gratified."[52]

All Because Eve Ate That Apple

This invocation of God punishing women may sound melodramatic. But religious disapproval lies at the origin of women's sexual self-loathing. The eighteenth-century ideal of desireless, anorgasmic women, after all, was a reaction against the opposing view: that women were insatiable, devious, and prone to sensual temptation. The temptation that made Eve eat from the tree of knowledge. To ensure women didn't cave to their impulses, church leaders denied these impulses' existence. It's almost as if we've assumed God made our orgasms elusive because our pleasure is wrong. First, women were cursed due to our aptitude for pleasure. Today, we are cursed for our supposedly low sexual capacity. While the myth itself has morphed, the curse has been carried down Eve's line from generation to generation.

Both these paradoxical condemnations of female sexuality affected Kaytlin. Even as she felt dysfunctional for *not* orgasming, she felt shame at the thought of enjoying sex. She believes this shame was behind her difficulty climaxing with partners: She'd suppressed her body's responses lest she appear too desirous or impure. "I was just like, 'oh my God, I'm so complicated, I'm so hard to make come that I must be super special,'" she muses. "I connected my inability to orgasm with a kind of sexual abstinence. I got the idea that withholding my orgasm, withholding my pleasure, was a form of not being a slut." She'd learned that since her "power" lay in men wanting sex more than her, she could control them by denying sex. She hadn't learned this would also require self-denial.

The irony is, despite the puritanical depiction of sexual pleasure as unwomanly, many women don't feel like themselves without it. "I got better at shaking those feelings of disappointment off, but they still deeply affected my self-esteem," says Margaret. Self-esteem is at the core of the matter, which is why this is about more than orgasms. When women learn they have less access to pleasure than men, they learn they have less of a *right* to pleasure. Not because their minds create that association, but because it's been there from the get-go. It's been there since the church feared and attempted to tamp down women's sexual urges. It's been there since scientists and politicians scrambled for evidence of women's inferiority. It's been there since physicians declared that women's role in sex and love was to please men or, at best, feel pleasure because of men. As long as we approach the orgasm gap from the biological perspective the two-sex model set in motion, inferiority complexes, devaluing, and shame will infiltrate women's bedrooms and undermine their sense of personhood. Soon, I'll turn to the new ways activists are tackling the orgasm gap and how Kaytlin, Margaret, and I unwound it in our own lives. But we have a few more old, heavy historical ruins to excavate first.

Chapter 6

PMS, from "a Raging Animal" to "Blood Coming Out of Her Wherever"

Meg Calvin used to spend a week in hell every month. "Before I would start bleeding, I would be really bloated and have a rollercoaster of emotions and breakouts and cramping," she recounts. "I was told 'that's just normal' and 'some women have it worse than others' by my doctor and other female voices in my life." Members of her church taught her that "pain as a woman has become our punishment for original sin" – the sin people are born with due to Adam and Eve's choice to eat from the tree of knowledge. They also claimed that "my period was a weakness because it would make me emotionally unstable," Meg recalls. As a result, she considered it unavoidable to be "easily offended," "easily triggered," and full of "intrusive anxious thoughts" premenstrually. She'd load up on Midol – the only solution her doctor offered – but her symptoms persisted.

The phenomenon Meg experienced is known as premenstrual syndrome, or PMS. The American College of Obstetricians and Gynecologists defines PMS as "physical or mood changes during the days before menstruation" that "happen month after month" and "affect a woman's normal life."[1] A meta-analysis of seventeen studies around the world found 48% of women report PMS symptoms, which range from breast tenderness to bloating to mood swings.[2] Between 5 and 8% of menstruators suffer from Premenstrual Dysphoric Disorder (PMDD), which is "similar to PMS but involves more severe symptoms, including depression, irritability, and tension, that impact a person's work or social functioning," according to the American Psychiatric Association.[3] But like the distinction between primary and secondary period pain, the distinction between PMS and PMDD may be misleading. It suggests the latter is a problem while the former is not. As it turns out, neither mild *nor* severe mental upset before one's period is normal. Like menstrual pain, PMS reflects underlying issues in women's lives and in society.

A Societal Syndrome

While it's easy to see PMS as a biological problem as old as Eve, the concept is recent. "PMS" came into common usage around the 1970s, as women were gaining status.[4] Like many scientific theories about women, it was tied to anti-feminist backlash, spawning "the cultural belief that women are erratic and unreliable" and legitimizing "attempts to restrict women's access to equal opportunities," Western Sydney University professors Jane Ussher and Janette Perz write in a paper in *Sex Roles*.[5] In 1970, American surgeon and politician Edgar Berman said women made poor leaders due to their "raging hormonal imbalances."[6] Four decades later, when Bill O'Reilly asked commentator Marc Rudov about the downsides of a female president in light of Hillary Clinton's campaign, Rudov replied: "You mean besides the PMS and the mood swings, right?"[7] When Clinton ran again in 2015, Texas CEO Cheryl Rios opined that "there's an old biblical sound reasoning why a woman shouldn't be president." That reasoning? "With the hormones we have, there is no way [a woman] should be able to start a war."[8]

Another favorite move for misogynists: invoking menstruation to discredit any and all points made by a woman during a disagreement. It's why Donald Trump's description of media personality Megyn Kelly – "there was blood coming out of her eyes, blood coming out of her wherever ... she was off base" – hit a nerve.[9] So many women have had men insinuate they were broken for bleeding, not just physically but psychologically. The curse is on the mind as much as the reproductive system. But *are* women cursed, or are they simply pointing out inconvenient truths? It's no coincidence that Trump's comment was spurred by Kelly's questions about his past sexist remarks. Hormones make for a handy rhetorical tool to diminish women's calls for equality.

The original concept of PMS was deeply intertwined with stereotypes of nagging, bitching women. Its precursor "premenstrual tension" was introduced in a 1931 paper by American gynecologist Robert Frank declaring some women prone to "foolish and ill-considered actions" right before their periods.[10] Later, in the 1953 *British Medical Journal* paper that coined the term "premenstrual syndrome," English physicians Raymond Greene and Katharina Dalton described symptoms women experienced "usually without complaining to their doctors but not necessarily without disturbing the tranquility of their homes."[11] The subsequent events that made PMS mainstream were even more enmeshed with ideas about women's out-of-control emotions. In the early 1980s, lawyers evoked the syndrome to exonerate two British criminals. Sandie Smith, who was charged with threatening a police officer, had already been convicted of multiple crimes including stabbing a coworker to death. Her attorney argued she couldn't help but turn into a "raging animal" each month due to PMS. The other woman, Christine English, fatally ran over a lover with her car. Her lawyer declared she suffered from "an extremely aggravated form of premenstrual physical condition," leading the judge to conclude she committed this act under "wholly exceptional circumstances" and reduce her charges from murder to manslaughter. The term "premenstrual syndrome" circulated in newspapers and magazines thereafter, solidifying perceptions of menstruators as unstable and untrustworthy.[12]

Is PMS Real?

Like period pain and painful sex, PMS is seen as a price women pay for being female. In one University of Massachusetts study, women called PMS "just a way of life for women" and "a side effect of menstruating."[13] But Sally King, research associate in menstrual physiology at King's College London, considers PMS a "cultural artifact." Despite nearly a century of research, no study has proven that hormonal shifts cause premenstrual mood fluctuations.[14] Such mood changes are not universal but reported primarily in Western Europe, Australia, and North America.[15] And frequently, so-called PMS stems from other conditions. The notion of PMS is "blaming emotional distress on the female body," King says. "'You're so upset and you're so angry at us and you're shouting at us because of your body! And you can't help it because of your body.' That is to completely undermine the experience of women and people who menstruate, which is usually pretty shitty. They just want to attribute women's distress to femininity – and certainly not the distressing things we experience."

Once again, our bodies are seen as the problem when the world around us is – and we're having valid reactions to it. Yet we are so constantly gaslit, we've come to gaslight ourselves. We internalize the derogatory messages around us. In one Mexican study, women who watched a video describing PMS reported more symptoms before their next period than those who watched a neutral video about the menstrual cycle. And the Massachusetts study found that women who subscribe to traditional femininity are more likely to report PMS.[16] They've learned women are emotional, so they dismiss their own emotions as feminine flaws. As women's health researcher Jane Ussher said on the *Hormonal* podcast:

> Women actually experience anger, depression, distress ... across the whole cycle. But what we know is that when they're premenstrual, they'll attribute it to their bodies, but when they're at other times of the cycle, they'll attribute it to other things in their life. So they might say, "oh, it's my partner" or "I'm late for work" or, you know, "it's Monday morning and I'm feeling lousy." So even within Western culture, we can see the way women are actually inculcated in what some might say is a negative discourse around menstruation.[17]

But it's not all in our heads. Mood changes can happen during the luteal phase – the two weeks or so before menstruation – for several reasons. One is that some women who report PMS are experiencing hormonal imbalances. Some of the same factors contributing to period pain also contribute to PMS. Research has linked PMS to deficiencies in calcium, magnesium, vitamin D, and B vitamins, as well as smoking, sugar, and processed foods.[18] Those who avoid hormone-disrupting chemicals, stay physically active, and have access to nature report lower PMS rates.[19] These same factors appear to be behind PMDD, further blurring this distinction.[20] And as usual, wider injustices are at play: Premenstrual symptoms have been linked to low socioeconomic class and education levels as well as stress and beauty norms. Some women who get bloated premenstrually report dips in mood due to feeling "fat" and self-conscious.[21]

Premenstrual symptoms can also be tied to underlying ailments, from mental illnesses like bipolar disorder to physical conditions like fibromyalgia and migraines. In these cases, PMS is a misnomer. A more accurate label is "premenstrual exacerbation," says King, as these patients are facing flareups of preexisting issues due to inflammation that occurs during the luteal phase. The period itself is not the problem; the untreated illness is. "Any kind of chronic health condition – most of those can be triggered by the menstrual cycle," King says. "It should not be mysterious: The immune system is highly inflammatory, so anything affecting immune responses is going to be triggered or worsened by the menstrual cycle." These patients experience health problems all month long, but their treatment is delayed by the perception that they're dealing with "normal" PMS. "Most of these people have very distressing behavior disruptive to their lives," says King. "We should talk to this person about what is upsetting them: When did this start? Are they experiencing something that's traumatic?" It's also possible menstruation isn't hurting these patients – the cycle's other phases are helping them. Estrogen, which rises after menstruation, alleviates anxiety and depression, King says, so some cases of "PMS" may be better dubbed "postmenstrual distress alleviation."

Unfortunately, PMS and PMDD's causes are poorly understood, thanks to the gendered research gap discussed in chapter 2. As of 2016, there were over five times more published studies on erectile dysfunction than PMS.[22] Scientists seem more keen on explaining PMS as a natural phenomenon. It's hypothesized that PMS evolved to make women reproduce with new mates out of rage toward their current partners, or that it's part of a hormonal cycle that encourages mating during the more fertile follicular phase.[23] These attempts to paint PMS as a blessing in disguise reinforce views of it as a curse. They suggest it's normal for women to be miserable for a quarter of their lives. As long as it helps them have babies!

Gaslighting Writ Large

Mental shifts throughout the cycle may not always indicate illnesses or imbalances. Estrogen and progesterone drop the week before your period, which some doctors say is behind premenstrual irritability.[24] Others, like nutritionist and menstrual activist Alisa Vitti, say a healthy cycle involves some mood shifts, but positive ones. For instance, someone experiencing a healthy luteal phase may want more space and set more boundaries but won't be cranky or testy.[25] The data is still up in the air, however, as to what role hormones play. "Everyone who menstruates experiences hormonal changes, and yet only some people experience PMS," says King. She finds it more likely that drops in mood stem from inflammation. Prostaglandins, the inflammatory compounds behind uterine contractions, rise during the luteal and menstrual phases.[26] As I discussed in chapter 1, debilitating inflammation isn't normal. But due to a host of factors from stress to undiagnosed illnesses, some deal with excessive prostaglandins and inflammation. And when someone's inflamed, their mental energy and patience diminish. Unsurprisingly, women with higher inflammation levels report more premenstrual mood symptoms.[27]

Some new age gurus speculate that premenstrual mood changes give women special intuitive powers. But King is skeptical of this, as beliefs in "female intuition" veer into "men are from Mars, women are from Venus" territory. I'm wary of this too, at least as a universal. Subscribers to this school of thinking have told me my emotions stemmed from the sacred luteal intuition when I was having justified reactions to something else entirely. This can feel just as dismissive, reductive, and presumptuous as when misogynists say it. Still, there's one kernel of truth to the idea that premenstrual feelings contain wisdom: Our emotions are valid even if they're influenced by hormones, inflammation, or whatever it is. Even those who are sensitive at this time are still sensitive *to* something. Often, the issues that come up premenstrually are issues women notice but stay silent about the rest of the month. Setting boundaries and expressing needs is healthy – and lots of women don't do it enough. As King puts it:

> Most of us have experienced things we'd normally put up with, and before our period, we're like, "I'm gonna tell this person they're really irritating." There's usually an external trigger. It's just that our body's busy, and we do have less tolerance. The pain is very real, but the social construction is very influenced by this idea that women are debilitated by their bodies.

Regardless of what's causing some women's heightened sensitivity, having a powered-up bullshit detector is not a bad thing. It shows someone what in their life needs changing. "I do recommend people take a note of what is pissing them off the most," says King. "For most people, it's their boss or their partner or a combination of things: You're working full-time but your partner doesn't do any of the childcare. Whatever it is you find most upsetting when you've got really low tolerance, it is worth doing something about that later on, when you feel a bit stronger. You can say: 'It's not because of my hormones; it's because I lose my ability to tolerate your lack of support.'"

Perhaps what really stands in the way of women's happiness during the luteal phase is the stigma against assertive women. If we valued women's voices, any extra attunement to mistreatment would be a good thing. After all, don't we want a world where women are treated better? Where the microaggressions women face can be spotted and prevented, no matter how small? Maybe some don't – and maybe that's why we're still stuck in stereotypes of premenstrual women as moody bitches rather than rightfully indignant. It's a convenient way to dismiss women's complaints rather than change what they're complaining about. Women's bullshit detectors are going off left and right because there is a lot of bullshit in this world. Women's bodies are shining light on it. It's up to us if we look or turn a blind eye.

On Estrogen and Emotionality

The truth is, women are no more hormonally driven than men. Sperm production involves cyclical changes in testosterone, luteinizing hormone, gonadotropin-releasing hormone, and follicle-stimulating hormone.[28] "The production of sperm from start to finish takes 2.5–3 months, but new sperm is initiated every thirteen days, so the process overlaps," King explains. "So super hormonal, yet nobody mentions men and their hormones." Men's testosterone levels also change throughout the day, starting off highest in the morning and dropping in the evening.[29] Testosterone, like any hormone, impacts mood, with rises contributing to anger in some situations.[30] Since men have more testosterone, it would be easy to dismiss them as hormonal. We don't, however, criticize men for being testosterone-pumped if they happen to be mad. We don't claim they can't hold office because they may have to make morning meetings when they're extra moody. And we take their anger seriously regardless of what their hormones are doing. After all, it's a reaction to real situations. So is women's anger, says King:

> If this was men and people said "we think the reason guys kill themselves more than women is that they get hangry because they have more muscle mass," we'd say, "What?" Testosterone is seen as great and estrogen is seen as worse, but men and women are as hormonal as each other. Hormones are nonstop components of the body's ecosystem. They go in and out all the time.

Ironically, women are accused of emotionality when their estrogen levels are lowest – most like men's. Estrogen drops during the late luteal phase and reaches its lowest point as menstruation starts.[31] As feminist activist Gloria Steinem pointed out: "If women are supposed to be less rational and more emotional at the beginning of our menstrual cycle when the female hormone is at its lowest level, then why isn't it logical to say that, in those few days, women behave the most like the way men behave all month long?"[32] Many stereotypes about hormones defy logic. Postmenopausal women have less estrogen than men their age – so are older men more emotional than their female peers?[33] Men who put down women's hormones are putting down their own biology – because the same hormones course through their veins.

Reframing the Luteal Phase

Another reason women may appear "hormonal" is that we believe they are. The way people see and treat menstruators affects their experiences of menstruation. This may be why premenstrual mood fluctuations aren't reported in all parts of the world. In Hong Kong, China, and India, where "menstruation is invariably positioned as a natural event," women "report premenstrual water retention, pain, fatigue, and increased sensitivity to cold, but rarely report negative premenstrual moods," write Ussher and Perz.[34] Some women only start to report PMS or PMDD after moving to the US or UK. When Ussher interviewed migrants and refugees in Australia about PMS, they gave responses like: "There isn't such a thing." When she asked Asian and Latin American women if they felt irritable before their periods, some said: "When I think about it, I do sometimes, but it's not a big deal."[35]

Other research confirms that premenstrual irritability is far from universal. In a review of forty-seven studies on mood throughout the cycle, only seven found mood changes specific to the premenstrual phase. Eighteen found no mood changes in any phase.[36] And only 12% of 2,900 women in one French study had moderate to severe PMS affecting their daily lives.[37] A higher number of women – two thirds in one University of Toronto study – report favorable premenstrual changes like heightened libido, productivity, energy, and creativity.[38] We rarely hear about these blessings thanks to the cultural curse on the luteal phase. A curse compounded by those who view women through its stigmatizing lens. In a study of sixty women with PMS, Ussher and Perz found that those in heterosexual relationships reported more premenstrual distress, depression, and anxiety than those in lesbian relationships because their male partners pathologized their feelings and withheld support.[39] A woman who starts off reasonably put off about something will become flat-out angry if a man refuses to listen. Then, there you go, PMS! Men who call women "crazy" could stand to examine the things they may be doing to make them that way – labeling them "crazy" being one of them.

It's not just external judgments that affect women's premenstrual emotions, but women's self-judgments. For Meg, unpacking negative views of menstruation was the first step toward eliminating the PMS that used to consume her life. She stopped minimizing the worries that came up before her period and began addressing them. She made time for self-care, avoided triggering situations, reduced her caffeine intake to balance her hormones, and took phase-specific dietary suggestions from Alisa Vitti's book *Woman Code* and app MyFLO.[40] Vitti tells me that when she works with women one-on-one to make lifestyle changes, it's common for their period issues to fade in a few cycles. "The intrusive anxious thoughts definitely decreased," says Meg. And her mood swings, bloating, and cramping went away. She's in the same body, but after reframing its phases, she experiences it differently. The funny thing is, she still gets some anxious thoughts before her period, but she's no longer troubled by them. Once she learned to prioritize self-care, fears that weren't grounded in reality fell away. Nowadays, her worries tend to point toward real issues in her life. If a concern is still there the week she starts bleeding, she concludes that "it's not just an anxious fear or a fantasy; it's something I need to take action on," she explains. "If I take care of my body and I'm letting myself sleep in and letting myself rest and letting myself be an introvert – as long as I'm gentle to myself – I can totally trust my feelings."

Dismantling the Myth of Menstrual Irrationality

As Meg's story shows, even if some women experience mental changes premenstrually, this doesn't make them irrational. In fact, a 2016 University College London study found that women's financial choices were just as rational as men's in every phase of their cycle.[41] And a 2017 University Hospital Zürich study found no correlation between women's cyclical hormonal changes and their performance on tasks testing attentiveness, memory, and self-control.[42] Even those who are about to have blood coming out of their "wherever" have capable brains.

Women who speak out about the problems around them often are dismissed as "PMSing." But women are not reactive to injustice because they're PMSing. It's the other way around. Much of what we call "PMS" is the body and mind launching a response to injustice. Our bodies are inflamed because society is not set up for our thriving. Our hearts are burning with anger because we have not been honored. We have been gaslit, invalidated, fragilized. We have had our feelings shoved under the rug. We have been told we're not enough and that we're too much. We have been poked and prodded at. For all this, we are angry, and this anger ends up leveraged as proof of our inferiority. But it is really proof our bodies know they were never meant to be put down. It is proof our hearts know they were never meant to be ignored. Ignoring women's feelings does a disservice to us all. It is by hearing our needs that we can create a world with less suffering. Not just premenstrually, but all month long. Not just for women, but for everyone.

Chapter 7

The Institutionalization of Sorrowful Childbirth

When Debra Pascali-Bonaro first got pregnant in Montreal, Canada in 1981, home births and midwife care were illegal. Her great grandma, who birthed all her kids at home, had taught her the importance of movement during labor. But it was standard for hospitals to use IVs and fetal monitoring that immobilized parents. So, a hospital birth was not Debra's top choice – but out of necessity, she searched for a hospital where she felt comfortable. "That wasn't easy," she remembers. "Everyone was pushing me to accept a medical model and wasn't listening to me. They didn't hear what my concerns were. They didn't validate that my birth was a natural process. They were seeing it through the lens of medicine. They were suggesting, 'Why don't you have an epidural?' I felt really disrespected and unheard and like I was just a young woman – what would I know compared to a physician's knowledge? I had to navigate through a broken system that was forcing me to give birth on my back." She finally found a student resident at a local medical school who OKed her giving birth upright without medication. But when she showed up for her birth, he wasn't there. She recalls:

The nurses belittled me. For a healthy, low-risk person, I felt they actually were going to put me at risk by overusing technology. I locked myself in the bathroom for a portion of my labor to avoid some of the common interventions. I came out when my doctor arrived, who I knew would listen to me. I was having to make sure that I created my own safety and said "no" to things that were stressful. Stress can make labor less enjoyable and more painful on every level: physical, emotional, and spiritual. I wanted what my great grandmother had: the joy and love that came from listening to her body and her baby.

The suffering involved in childbirth may seem like a biological inevitability if not a divine punishment. Yet like menstrual pain, painful sex, and PMS, it has been societally sanctioned and cemented. The very view of childbirth pain as punishment makes it appear an inevitability. Is it either? Our bodies hold the potential for painful labor, but also for much more. Cultural practices around childbirth, however, lead us down the path of pain and sometimes trauma. Once again, it is not divinity or biology but humanity that's seen women as physically defective – then treated them that way. So much so that our defectiveness appears like a scientific fact and everyday reality.

Thou Shalt Have Children in Fear

The religious view of childbirth as punishment isn't just inaccurate – it may not even be biblical. The normalization of labor pain is based more on debatable translations of the Bible than the original text. The popular New International Version says God told Eve: "I will make your pains in childbearing very severe; with painful labor you will give birth to children." In the classic King James Bible, the curse goes: "I will greatly multiply thy sorrow and thy conception; in sorrow thou shalt bring forth children." Most versions include "pain."[1] But J. Harvey Walton, a Bible scholar who wrote his PhD thesis on Genesis at the University of St. Andrews, thinks these translations miss the mark. The Hebrew word translated as "bring forth children" or "give birth to children," "yalad," describes the general experience of having kids more than the specific process of childbirth. Terms for labor pain like "chuwl" and "tsiyr" are absent from Adam and Eve's story. And the words translated to "pain" and "sorrow" – "'itstsâbôwn" and "ʽetseb" – mean "anxiety" or "mental and emotional distress," says Walton. So, a better translation might be "thou shalt reproduce anxiously" or "thou shalt have children in fear." Walton elaborates:

> I don't think that's the physical process. I think that's the anxiety associated with fertility and successful procreation. If you can't reproduce, it means your family line ends, and that means different things depending who you are. If you're a woman and you can't reproduce, that's grounds for divorce. That's grounds for lower status in your household. That's a threat to existence in the community. That's very scary. If you're a male, you need to continue your family's legacy because inheritance and everything else is patrilineal – so your entire extended family is counting on you to keep the property in your family.[2]

And if you're a woman who reproduces outside marriage – or is sexual enough to provoke fears that you might – this is grounds for shaming and exile. Which brings us back to the theory I put forth in chapter 1: The so-called curse in Genesis was a foretelling of humanity's transition from foraging to farming – the point in history when women's reproduction came under public control. Women's sexuality was monitored to ensure fathers could keep track of which children belonged to them. And so the "sorrow" and "anxiety" of bringing kids into the world could be paternity anxiety – and the broader fear of female freedom it spawned. This fear is behind many modern injustices: Slut shaming. Infringements upon reproductive justice. The Madonna-whore complex. Stigma against the child-free. And a childbirth system that silences women. Yes, "thou shalt have children in fear" was an accurate prediction. It foreshadowed the oppression women face. It's not Eve's choice to eat the apple that is making us suffer, but the mistreatment of her descendants because of it.

How Eve's Fall Became Women's Defectiveness

Ayelet Polonsky knew when she got pregnant that she wanted a home birth. While she was lucky enough to find a midwife who was on board, her friends made comments like "oh my gosh, I could never do that, you're crazy." There were "healthcare providers that tried to instill their views and tell me, 'You might want to consider giving birth at a hospital,'" she recalls. "I was like, they're allowed to have opinions and do things in what they think is the right way, but I'm also going to do things in what I think is the right way for me and my family. For me, not having someone tell me when to push, not having someone tell me that I might need a C-section or that they may need to use pliers to pull out the baby's head – I didn't want any intervention, and I didn't want anybody telling me what my body knows how to do."

Today, women's reproductive anxiety stems not just from the threat of being deemed infertile or unfaithful but from doctors, friends, and family worrying their bodies are incapable. The supposed curse is not just pain but incompetence, necessitating reliance on a patriarchal system. Unnecessary, harmful, and sometimes non-consensual interventions characterize the childbirth process throughout the Western world, with insurance coverage and social convention skewed toward hospital births.[3] While hospital births *should* be an option for safety's sake, the modern approach is not motivated solely by safety. As usual, ancient assumptions have snuck into ostensibly objective institutions.[4]

Giving birth at home was the standard in the US up until the early twentieth century, and the subsequent transition to hospitals was intertwined with notions of female inferiority. In a 1908 paper, Harvard doctor Franklin S. Newell advocated C-sections and forceps for upper-class women engaged in intellectual pursuits, claiming overuse of the mind hindered the reproductive system. Since their bodies were incapable, women required physicians' assistance.[5] Male doctors usurped midwives in the 1920s as factories boomed and childbirth took on an assembly line structure, transporting patients between hospital rooms at peak efficiency.[6] But myths of female defectiveness shaped childbirth long before then, leading to under-use of medicine prior to the age of over-medicalization. In the sixteenth century, midwives were penalized for offering pain relief, lest they defy God's command of sorrowful childbirth. One was burned at the stake for doing so.[7]

Today, both ideologies come into play. Some women are infantilized by providers over-intervening in their births, while others who choose interventions are judged for bypassing the supposedly necessary pain of labor. While all freely chosen settings can foster a healthy birth, neither of these attitudes does. The real debate is not between hospital and home births but between valuing women's voices and upholding their suffering.

When Healing Does Harm

Midwife Barbara Montani is still haunted by births she witnessed while working in Scottish and Italian hospitals. There, midwives made comments that depicted labor pain as punishment. "You hear 'well you know, you enjoyed getting the baby in, so now time to get the baby out' – like childbirth is a punishment for sex," she recalls. "The idea of pleasure being a sin that therefore you have to pay for is a very strong concept. And I feel like it's quite common in other religions as well that you somehow need to pay for the pleasure. It's like they want you to be in pain during labor. The system as a whole seems to encourage this concept of it having to be painful and degrading and humiliating. When Eve gets told 'you will give birth in pain,' it's almost like they revel in that; they want that to be the case."

Montani has seen doctors deny women pain relief they requested, with some hospitals only offering epidurals – the most common labor pain medication – from 8 a.m. to 8 p.m. Monday to Friday. On the flip side, she's witnessed non-consensual exams and procedures; she remembers one woman screaming "stop" as a doctor inserted an unneeded urinary catheter. While these two types of mistreatment fall on opposite ends of the spectrum of involvement, they stem from the same assumption of female defectiveness. The neglect for women's comfort and the imposing of unneeded comfort measures both reflect the normalization of suffering. Either women's pain is deemed unworthy of attention, or interventions are pushed on them because their pain and weakness are assumed. Episiotomies, where a doctor cuts tissue between the vagina and anus, are sometimes performed without consent under the belief that this helps get the baby out and prevent tearing.[8] But the body usually gets the baby out on its own, and natural tears heal faster than episiotomy cuts.[9] To advocate for herself and let her doctor know she accepted the risk of natural tears, Debra told him: "If you cut me, I'll cut you." Montani explains: "We've all seen episiotomies with little to no consent – with 'oh, I'm just gonna give you a little bit of a cut.' No, that is a procedure that requires you to gain informed consent." C-sections and medication for induction also get utilized without permission, Montani adds:

I witnessed the abuse of medical induction of labor – inducing labor when there is no medical reason to – all without informed consent. They just tell women they're getting induced, and they don't explain the induction process to them. The same with offering cesarean sections with little to no indication and women being told "it's best if we go for a C-section" when in actuality, a lot of the time, if you just let them be and don't interfere and spoil a perfectly good process, you wouldn't have had to go for a section in the first place. A lot of the time, it's like, "She's never gonna deliver that baby on her own; they need to induce labor." And induction of labor when needed is a great tool to have. But the overuse definitely ties into this concept of "women are incapable." Cesarean section as well ties into this bigger concept of women being incapable of giving birth on their own – of birth being an inherently dangerous and risky process rather than a natural phenomenon that will *sometimes* require medical intervention.

C-sections constitute 32% of births in the US – and over 50% in Brazil, the Dominican Republic, Cyprus, Egypt, and Turkey. Yet research finds that offering C-sections in over 15% of births offers no benefit for mothers or babies and actually has a net negative impact.[10] Some studies have correlated high C-section rates with complications and deaths due to the procedure's risks, which include immune, metabolic, and respiratory conditions in infants along with hemorrhage and infection in parents.[11] A 2019 study of over 3.5 million births in California found that parents who got C-sections had 2.7 times the risk of life-threatening complications during delivery.[12] Another study in France found that C-sections posed an 80% higher risk of severe complications than vaginal births.[13] The US maternal mortality rate more than quadrupled from 1987 to 2021, giving the US the highest rate of any developed country despite all the interventions used – or perhaps because of them.[14] The country's cesarean rate grew six-fold between 1970 and 2016.[15]

Putting Parents on Their Backs

The problem is not the existence of interventions but the lack of agency afforded in hospitals. "Our medical system saves lives, and it's a really needed resource when someone has a risk factor in pregnancy or birth," says Debra, now the doula trainer behind the *Orgasmic Birth* book and documentary. "A small percentage of people need additional technology. But by fully medicalizing birth, I believe we've done more harm than good. And part of that harm is we literally and figuratively put people down on their backs. We put people down emotionally. We don't set them up for wellness. Most people don't have a room with lots of options for comfort. Many hospitals use the same room for a sick person as a person giving birth – and that environment actually creates more pain, creates more labors that are self-fulfilling." In a 2024 study, one in seven people who gave birth in the US – including a quarter of LGBTQ parents – said they'd been mistreated during childbirth. The most common mistreatments were neglect, yelling, scolding, and threats.[16] Over a quarter of women in one Swiss study said they'd faced coercion from providers during childbirth.[17] Such treatment can mark the difference between a joyful birth and a sorrowful one. Women list control over their bodies and environments among the biggest factors facilitating positive births, with caregiver support and maternal decision-making power influencing birth satisfaction more than pain management.[18]

Some view birthing outside a hospital as naive given that many died in labor before hospitals became the go-to settings. However, the issue was never a lack of hospitals but a lack of competent attendance, says Montani. Infant death rates are slightly higher for home and midwife center births than hospital births, but they're low for both (3.9 vs. 1.8 per 1,000 births, according to an Oregon study), and babies are less likely to end up in the intensive care unit after out-of-hospital births.[19] For low-risk mothers, there are only 4.3 adverse outcomes for the baby per 1,000 births whether they're in midwife units or obstetric units, according to an Oxford University study of over 64,000 births in England.[20] And those who birth at midwife centers or at home utilize fewer interventions, which can cause complications and reduce birth satisfaction. "The results support a policy of offering healthy women with low-risk pregnancies a choice of birth setting," the Oxford study concluded.[21] The goal is not to eradicate any approach but to decipher which approaches work best for which births. Through individualized care, we can allow the automatic childbirth process to take place but intervene when necessary, balancing security and sovereignty.

This balance should exist for postpartum care as well, which suffers from the opposite problem. Despite medical providers' high involvement in childbirth, parents are often left without support afterward. US companies are required to offer just three months of unpaid leave, contributing to postpartum depression, job loss, and even infant and child mortality.[22] Adam's curse is Eve's. The mandate that we painfully toil makes having children a sorrowful experience. And it is not just sexism but racism and colonialism that cause this pain. Our work-focused Western value system has overridden Indigenous practices that celebrate and pamper parents.[23] As the terms "'itstsâbôwn" and "'etseb" suggest, emotional pain characterizes modern childbirth. The soullessness with which we approach labor makes it all that much more painful.

The Cycle of Fear and Pain

When people have children anxiously, this has physical consequences. Fear leads to tension, which leads to pain. If someone is anxious during labor, their pelvis clenches, their blood flow is restricted, and stress hormones called catecholamines rise. This physical response can decrease mobility, cause discomfort, and slow or stop labor.[24] As Debra describes her first birth: "I think more of the pain was fear – fear that I wasn't being treated right. Because I found less pain in subsequent births. I don't think the pain on a physical level gets less. I don't think I was supported, so because I was tense, because I was afraid, it felt harder on every level. We have pain on an emotional and physical level. I think that existed on all levels in that first birth. In subsequent births, I feel like I had that support. I certainly didn't have emotional stress or pain. So it was more manageable to have intensity. I wouldn't even call it pain in my third birth."

Typically during labor, a hormone called oxytocin stimulates contractions and "tells your brain to produce endorphins, which we know are the brain's own natural painkiller," Montani says. "And the production of your own endorphins then stimulates even more oxytocin to be produced. So if you are able to create that feedback system, that is where you see that beautiful labor zone of the woman being completely zoned out and doing her own thing." But stress interrupts the hormonal processes necessary for a healthy delivery, and some medical environments unfortunately cause stress, says Montani: "Brightly lit hospital rooms full of strangers, painful procedures ... all that scares the oxytocin away and therefore scares the endorphins." This hormonal deficit not only enables pain but impedes labor – so, to jump-start labor, a synthetic oxytocin called Pitocin may be administered. Pitocin is notorious for inducing intense contractions. "People don't feel safe; they don't feel respected, and so these hormones, which are shy, don't flow," Debra explains. "So we use synthetic oxytocin and medications and drugs and are making labor more painful." If someone finds Pitocin-induced contractions unbearable, they may request an epidural – a medication that numbs you from the waist down – which can further inhibit oxytocin, make it hard to push, and necessitate instruments like forceps and vacuums. These instruments in turn increase the risk of tears and urinary incontinence.[25] This is one example of what birth workers call the "cascade of interventions," where medical interventions create problems requiring more interventions, which in turn create more problems.

The cycle of fear and pain is even more insidious for survivors of sexual and medical trauma, including previous traumatic births. Survivors can experience flashbacks when doctors silence their voices, make choices without their consent, and undermine their bodies' capabilities.[26] Invasive, non-consensual exams and procedures can themselves be traumatic. Even without this, birth can bring violations experienced in past healthcare settings to the surface. For instance, it's legal in many US states for medical students to perform pelvic exams on women put under for unrelated procedures without their knowledge.[27] If someone has gone through this, the loss of control during childbirth can be terrifying, and the body may clench to protect itself. The cycle of tension and pain continues, not just for individuals but for a medical system that responds to pain with fear and to fear with measures that cause more pain.

This cycle makes the expectation of sorrowful birth self-fulfilling. The tales about birth's terrors may build up tension as someone anticipates their delivery date. Those who have more fear and expect more pain in childbirth end up experiencing more pain.[28] "We live in a fear-based society," Ayelet observes. "People have this notion that labor is what they see in movies, with women in a hospital bed screaming their lungs out and it's a big bloody mess. That's not necessarily the case." Nineteen percent of women report less pain than expected during birth, and only 45% describe their pain as a negative experience. Many master it: Under 2% of those who birth at home get transferred to the hospital for pain relief.[29] And if we encouraged less fear and treated parents with more dignity, childbirth pain would be less severe and common. In a study of twenty-one Australian women, those who practiced mindful acceptance found birth sensations more manageable than those who were "distracted and distraught." One frequent source of distraction and distress was providers telling mothers they were running into problems or not progressing as hoped.[30] When women receive the message that their bodies are cursed, their births adhere to this limiting narrative.

How Social Injustice Spawns Sorrowful Childbirth

Due to the downsides of hospital births, more people are giving birth in their homes or midwife centers. But these options are often inaccessible. As of 2024, thirteen US states don't license professional midwives. So midwives work in a legal gray area, lacking access to lab tests and medications.[31] Even after rising by 12% from 2020 to 2021, home births still constituted only 1.41% of US births.[32] Just around .5% of births take place at midwife centers.[33] And it is mostly White Americans who evade hospitals, which are especially hostile toward people of color. Black women in the US are 2.6 times as likely as White women to die from pregnancy or childbirth.[34] Native Americans' maternal mortality rate is similarly twice as high as White Americans'.[35] This discrepancy stems from medical racism as well as disparities in hospital quality. In hospitals that disproportionately treat Black patients, birthers face more complications like pulmonary embolisms when they hemorrhage – that is, bleed due to damaged blood vessels.[36]

Meanwhile, alternatives like midwife care are White-dominated and not always in reach. Eighty-six percent of US midwives are now White even though 73% were Black from 1880 to 1930.[37] "As birth left the home and began to occur in hospitals, White male doctors understood that to make their money, they had to take birth out of the home – and put all these prerequisites in place that put Black midwives out of business," explains birth doula Ngozi Tibbs. The field of gynecology, in fact, was founded through dangerous experiments on slaves, which affects how Black women are treated in medical settings today.[38] In a 2016 study, half of White medical students and residents endorsed false beliefs about racial differences such as "Black people's nerve endings are less sensitive than White people's nerve endings" and "Whites, on average, have larger brains than Blacks."[39] As a result, Black women's pain gets doubly dismissed and treated as a spectacle.

For Tanisha Bowman, a mother in Pittsburgh, PA, this bias was hard to deny. Right after giving birth, she began having bladder spasms, and blood showed up in her urine. Hospital staff members gathered around her, and one said: "You would make an interesting paper." It turned out she had a bladder full of blood clots, but providers' lack of empathy delayed this diagnosis. "I was horrified; that sticks with me forever," she recalls. "It took them forever to show up, and all of a sudden, there's a room full of White people looking at me – not telling me what's wrong with me, but telling me how interesting the case was. And I'm sitting there like, 'Am I about to die?'" They then brought her to the intensive care unit, where she was left alone while her child went home. "I lost my mind," she recalls. "I wasn't attended to, and I didn't feel comfortable complaining because I didn't want to be that patient people were annoyed by. I remember neuro coming in and taking one look at me like I was a mess and running out the door and not even communicating with me. There's a vulnerability in that bed that people don't appreciate until they're in that bed. I needed care. I needed help. But I was afraid because I've witnessed the snarkiness of staff toward patients who seem too needy."

After leaving with a walker and catheter, Tanisha had nightmares about her time in the hospital. "I was having intrusive thoughts," she says. "I would be afraid that I was going to drop the car seat when we were going up the stairs." These are signs of postpartum PTSD, something 22% of parents – including over 36% of Black parents – meet at least some criteria for. Black mothers are at especially high risk if they're deprived of autonomy and disrespected by providers.[40] LGBTQ parents are also vulnerable to birth trauma, as providers disrespect their identities and family structures.[41] Shanéa from chapter 4 recalls "walking out upset" after medical staff made assumptions about him and his transmasculine partner: "They'd misgender me or say something weird. I was like, we don't need to do this. I just need my checkup." As a doula, Ngozi had to call out nurses for whispering about how her lesbian client may have conceived. "I was like, am I curious? Sure," she says. "But I'm not going to ask that because that's invasive. What's most important is that we respect people's humanity." Fatphobia enters childbirth settings, too. During one of her own births, Ngozi grew frightened when she needed medication for high blood pressure, and the nurse said she'd tolerate it fine because she was "big." Ngozi recalls: "I felt embarrassed. I had to open my legs to this woman."

It is such treatment that truly makes childbirth full of anguish. We cannot talk about suffering in birth without acknowledging injustices toward marginalized parents. We cannot talk about labor pain without talking about invalidation and infantilization. Parents do not need providers to save them from their own bodies. They need a support system that works with their bodies and helps them trust themselves.

The Ultimate Gift

Some may wonder: Does the fact that our healthcare system makes childbirth *more* painful negate that it *is painful*? Childbirth is the ultimate sacrifice, after all; don't women deserve credit for all they go through? I'll circle back to this question in chapter 13, which shares the experiences of women who indeed gave birth painlessly. After hearing and reading dozens of pleasurable birth stories, the most common description I've come across is that these births were intense but not painful. Some describe fleeting moments of pain, which signal a need to move, breathe, or change position to clear the way for comfort again. I've also heard stories from women who experienced *pain* but not *suffering* in childbirth, as it is often fear, trauma, and lack of support that escalate pain to the point of suffering.

Childbirth certainly is painful when it doesn't take place under the right circumstances, and later, we'll get into what those circumstances are. Someone's birth is not entirely under their control, and if situations arise that cause pain, that's not their fault. Especially if they belong to a marginalized group or lack access to attentive providers. I read the female body as a cipher, reflecting problems with how society treats women and everyone.[42] Women's bodily experiences are feedback about the world around them, and right now, we live in a world where people don't listen to women – or encourage women to listen to themselves. Because of that, most births are painful, and that will not change overnight. It will require a cultural move toward gender equality, sexual liberation, medical reform, and economic access. Yet I believe that ultimately, it's possible to set up a society where pain during birth is not the norm.

What happens then? If parents don't suffer through childbirth, will we have less reason to revere them? I don't think so. Even pain-free births require strength and fortitude – and finding pleasure is itself worthy of reverence. We must let go of our "no pain, no gain" mentality to see that childbirth is just as honorable without discomfort. "I see labor as an opportunity to bring more light into the world through my vessel, and what a gift," says Ayelet. What if we revered childbirth not as the ultimate sacrifice, but as the ultimate gift? A gift to the child, the family, the community, and the world – but also to the mother. A gift we will be robbed of as long as we equate womanhood with sacrifice.

Chapter 8

Trauma: An Assault on the Body

Josefina Bashout describes her early childhood as a journey from "riches to rags." When she was nine, her parents divorced and her father moved back to his home country of Egypt, leaving her mother and their six kids in poverty in Los Angeles. Soon after, when Josefina was in sixth grade, her mom's boyfriend violently molested her then threw a $5 bill at her, as if to designate this was all she was worth. Due to his physical and sexual abuse, she entered the foster care system and had to testify in court at age twelve. Constantly moving between families and schools, she didn't have people around for support, so she bottled up her feelings. "My sexual molestation experience shut me down and had me detach from my body as a coping mechanism," she remembers.

She experimented with masturbation as a teenager, but she felt uneasy and had, at most, "baby orgasms" she could barely feel. "I couldn't really feel in my body – it was more numb than sensations and not really much pleasure," she says. "I didn't really have a full orgasm. I'd get to a point, then I'd feel all this pressure, then I'd get scared and be like, 'Now, I'm done.'" In her twenties, she built up a career in the product development industry, working with celebrity clients. But outside work, she numbed herself with alcohol and partying. She had unfulfilling sex with actors and models just to prove she could earn their attention, coasting by high off the thrill of her professional accomplishments and Hollywood parties. After one partner gave her her first real orgasm, she began reading about sexuality and exploring it more consciously.

Then, she became involved with a man who took issue with her growing interest in sex. He called her a "slut" and "whore" for being "too open" sexually. Meanwhile, he secretly used live sex chat rooms that fetishized Middle Eastern women like her. She remembers dressing in a sexy outfit for him on Valentine's Day, only for him to lash out. His abuse escalated to the point that he physically attacked her for touching a male friend's chest at a party, then carried her TV out of her apartment while announcing it was "worth more than her," triggering flashbacks of that $5 bill. "I was inside to deal with myself, and I was so devastated and so distraught and felt so unsafe and had been in an abusive situation, which I now know was generational – my mom was in an abusive relationship and marriage," she says. "I was repeating a generational pattern in my lineage of women who are submissive and who are in these toxic, abusive relationships where their sexuality is shamed, where their expression is shamed."

A month later, she went to the doctor for a well-woman exam, and he mentioned her pap smear appeared abnormal. After further labwork, she received an unsettling piece of news: She'd tested positive for HPV and severe high-grade pre-cervical cancer. This "was a huge wakeup call of: you're disconnected," she remembers. "Your body's yelling, she's speaking, she's crying." She believes her cervix was reacting not just to the abuse she herself survived, but to a larger culture that keeps women afraid and uncomfortable in their bodies.

The Impact of Rape Culture, Down to Our Cells

The awareness of this larger culture is only in its infancy. Until five decades ago in US history, sexual assault and intimate partner violence were considered isolated occurrences rather than a society-wide epidemic. Feminists began busting this myth in the 1970s, with the term "rape culture" introduced in 1974's *Rape: The First Sourcebook for Women* by activists Noreen Connell and Cassandra Wilson.[1] A year later, Susan Brownmiller's *Against Our Will: Men, Women, and Rape* described the "rape-supportive culture" throughout the US and the world, calling rape "a conscious process of intimidation by which *all men* keep *all women* in a state of fear."[2] The 1975 documentary *Rape Culture* spread this idea, demonstrating how the media normalizes sexual violence, from *Last Tango in Paris* and *Gone With the Wind* to men's magazines, and how social standards of masculinity encourage mistreatment of women.[3]

Recent statistics support activists' hypothesis that sexual trauma is a feature of modern society, not a bug. The World Health Organization estimates that one in three women worldwide will experience sexual violence or physical intimate partner violence in her lifetime.[4] Even this number may be low due to limited definitions of sexual violence. A 2019 survey of 182,000 American university students found that 39% of women and 40% of trans, non-binary, and genderqueer people had experienced non-consensual sexual contact – including rape and unwanted touching – during college alone.[5] Just as sexual assault was once viewed as an individual problem rather than a collective one, women's physical and mental illnesses often are now. Perhaps one day, women's health crises will be seen how their sexual trauma currently is, as understanding grows that the two are intertwined. When we consider how sexual violence impacts the victim's health, it becomes clear that sexual assault is an assault on the body. On the well-being of women and other marginalized people everywhere.

Josefina believes the trauma she endured in childhood had been stored in her cervix, tracing her illness to "the shame around my body, my physical abuse, that experience of seeing myself as unworthy." Supporting her theory, research has shown sexual abuse survivors are at high risk of cervical cancer and other pelvic conditions.[6] One 60,000-woman study found survivors of severe, chronic childhood physical and sexual abuse were 79% more likely to suffer from endometriosis.[7] Women with interstitial cystitis are 1.7 times as likely as symptom-free women to have been sexually abused.[8] IC patients who have survived sexual assault experience more tenderness during pelvic exams, as trauma can make the pelvic floor over-active and the nervous system hyper-responsive to pain. They also fare worse in all domains of sexual functioning.[9]

In unwinding my own bladder pain, I worked with a physical therapist who helped loosen my pelvic floor. She noticed I had tight muscles, which could have contributed to the discomfort on top of my UTI. I realized this muscle tightness had impeded my ability to feel pleasure as well as comfort. After treating it, orgasms felt more like they were right on the surface, not somewhere deep I had to dig for. It's unclear if my own pelvic pain was linked to sexual trauma. After all, I hadn't endured a major trauma like a rape. Just smaller incidents: strangers groping me on trains and at parties, hookup partners pressuring me to go further than I wanted, internet trolls messaging me with appearance-based insults and graphic descriptions of sex acts. This was how it was for Sophie too. "I never really labeled myself someone who had sexual trauma," she says. "It was more the little things that happened, but looking back, they were not really little because they had a big impact on how safe I feel in my body."

My favorite definition of trauma is psychologist Peter Levine's: It's "what we hold inside in the absence of an empathetic witness."[10] Rape culture deprives women of empathetic witnesses. It inundates us with bodily violations and minimizes them until we see them as "little things." Yet their impact on our well-being is big. Within rape culture, even everyday encounters seen as "normal" involve breaches of consent. Sophie's first time having intercourse resided in this middle ground between assault and consensual sex. She met a man in a bar, and after a few drinks, he "pushed himself" on her. "All of a sudden, I was like 'wow, there's a penis inside of me,'" she recalls. "I didn't even really know what was happening." Following that experience, Sophie continued having encounters born more from partners' desires than hers. She didn't know what else sex could look like. "That set the tone for me not having my own say in sex and not being connected to my 'yes' or my 'no,'" she says. "My body lost trust because I didn't really honor my boundaries. I didn't even know what they were."

Self-Protection and Sexual Shut-Down

When your earliest sexual experiences are non-consensual or halfheartedly consented to, you don't get the chance to associate sex with pleasure, respect, and happiness. A 2018 review of studies on sexual abuse survivors' sex lives concluded that this lack of positive associations leads to arousal problems.[11] If our experiences with intimacy are damaging or frightening, the body and mind are less apt to get excited in sexual situations. Encounters meant to bring joy and calm and bonding instead set off the brain's alarm system. On top of this, the mechanisms people develop to avoid uncomfortable emotions stemming from trauma dull pleasure. One University of Vermont study linked substance abuse, dissociation, and emotional suppression due to childhood sexual abuse with difficulty orgasming.[12] Given the prevalence of sexual trauma, it's no wonder 11–41% of women worldwide struggle to climax.[13]

Sophie believes her inability to orgasm with partners, even later ones she felt more comfortable with, stemmed from stuffing down her feelings. Because she'd blocked out the warning signals her body emitted during experiences she felt ambivalent about, she also ended up blocking out pleasure. "The longer I didn't really listen to my body because I didn't know how, the more my body shut down as a way to protect myself because I didn't even have a strong 'no' – I didn't know what that felt like," she says. Even though she grew up with a progressive family, nobody taught her what it meant to consent to sex. She knew it was assault if someone said "no," but she wasn't aware true consent meant expressing an enthusiastic "yes."

Even as laws pass in the US, Australia, and Europe defining consent by a "yes" rather than a lack of "no," public understanding is still catching up.[14] Only ten US states require that sex ed even teach consent.[15] In a 2015 survey, one in five Americans said someone was consenting if they didn't say "no." Just as many thought foreplay was consent for sex.[16] In another survey of 3,000 Australians ages twelve to twenty-four, a quarter considered it normal for men to pressure women into sex.[17] "Having sex when I didn't feel ready, I just thought that was normal," echoes Sophie. "I just thought that was what you were supposed to do." Yet the body doesn't treat this as normal. Sophie remembers instances where sex would become painful because her muscles would tense up. Since a trauma survivor's brain can treat sex as a threat, vaginal clenching becomes a defense. Vaginismus – involuntary vaginal tightening that makes penetration painful – is most common in sexual and emotional abuse survivors.[18]

Threat is far from an emotion one would hope to feel during intimacy, yet this feeling dominates many encounters. Multiple times when Kaytlin was in college, men surreptitiously removed condoms in the middle of sex without her knowledge. This was one reason she didn't orgasm with partners until her thirties: She became hyper-vigilant during sex. If she could remain aware of her surroundings at all times, she figured, no violation would escape her notice. "I started preventing myself from experiencing pleasure," she explains, "because getting into that headspace where I could really let go and enjoy the sex felt like I was too vulnerable." The phenomenon she experienced, dubbed "stealthing" in online communities where men teach the practice, is astoundingly common. In a study of 1,200 female visitors to an Australian sexual health clinic, 32% had experienced it.[19] Most unsurprisingly felt stressed as a result. "Having somebody I had consented to engage in protected sex with slipping the condom off – and these guys thought nothing of that – it was infuriating," Kaytlin remembers. Yet she found herself wondering if she was over-reacting. When she kicked one man out of her apartment, he yelled, "Woah, what's the big deal, jeez." In that moment, she felt like the crazy one.

Women: "Crazy" or Traumatized?

Rape culture is designed to make women feel "crazy" and wrong for not accepting sexual violence. And the stereotype of the crazy woman extends beyond such situations. It gets thrown around to discount women's voices and shame them for asserting needs, from PMS stereotypes to judgment of assertive women in the workplace. But *are* women mentally unstable? On the surface, statistics may appear to depict women as wired for mental illness. Globally, almost twice as many women as men meet the criteria for anxiety disorders. Major depressive disorder, bipolar II disorder, anorexia, and bulimia are more common in women.[20] Yet research has failed to find gender-based differences in emotional reactivity. In one University of Maryland study, men and women exhibited comparable changes in heart rate, blood pressure, and other measures of emotionality as they recalled events from their lives.[21] A University of Michigan study that had people record their emotions for seventy-five days found that women's did not fluctuate more than men's.[22] Men and women rate their feelings as similarly intense while they are feeling them. It's only in retrospect, once biases have the chance to creep in, that women sometimes rate theirs as stronger.[23] So, it's not that women respond more emotionally to the same circumstances as men. Perhaps it's that they're put into more maddening circumstances.

Sex and gender-diverse people are subject to similar assumptions of mental instability. A psychiatrist once suggested to Ed that he was trans *because of* PTSD from a sexual assault. Trans people do disproportionately face mental illness, but likely because they are also disproportionately trauma survivors. Forty-seven percent of trans and non-binary Americans have been sexually assaulted, and 54% have experienced harassment in K-12 settings alone.[24] And then there is the trauma simply of being looked down upon for your gender. Yet mental illness does not appear to cause or stem from trans-ness itself. Trans youth who are accepted by their peers have typical self-worth and depression rates.[25] What's really happening when women and sex and gender-diverse people are "crazy" or "unstable" is, often, they are experiencing the impact of trauma. Mental illness is not just one possible response to sexual violence – it's the typical one. Eighty percent of teenage girls who have been sexually assaulted meet the diagnostic criteria for at least one mental health disorder, and 55% meet the criteria for at least two.[26] These effects can follow someone for a lifetime: Adult survivors disproportionately face anxiety, depression, eating disorders, PTSD, sleep disorders, and suicide attempts.[27]

Even without a full-blown mental illness, the aftermath of sexual violence is stressful at the least – and chronic stress alone sets people up for physical and mental health issues down the line.[28] One can hear the distress in victims' testimonies. "I tried to push it out of my mind, but it was so heavy," Chanel Miller, who was sexually assaulted at a Stanford University party, said in her 2016 court statement. "I didn't interact with anyone. After work, I would drive to a secluded place to scream." Her memoir *Know My Name* describes her physical health impacted in ways that have ripple effects: "My basic functions began to falter: I stopped sleeping, forgot to eat, couldn't even shit properly."[29]

"When the sexual assault happened, I was a young woman brimming with confidence and looking forward to a future bright with possibilities," Andrea Constand, one of over sixty women to accuse Bill Cosby of assault, said in her victim impact statement. "Now, almost fifteen years later, I'm a middle-aged woman who's been stuck in a holding pattern for most of her adult life, unable to heal fully or to move forward." We won't get to hear the stories of every survivor like Miller, Constand, Josefina, Ed, and Kaytlin. But they're five of many, many people living in the aftermath of sexual violence. These survivors must contend not just with the incident but with the fallout that follows – one full of victim-blaming, shaming, and doubting from the legal system and sometimes their loved ones. Constand described feeling "traumatized all over again" when she faced her perpetrator in court. "I had to watch Cosby make jokes and attempt to degrade and diminish me, while his lawyers belittled and sneered at me. It deepened my sense of shame and helplessness, and at the end of each day, I left emotionally drained and exhausted."[30] It's not surprising many survivors of such crimes go on to struggle with mental health.

The Ultimate Invalidating Environment

Even if they escape assault, almost every woman experiences sexual harassment. Surveys in countries all over the world, from Latin America to the Middle East, show that the majority of women have been harassed. Eighty-six percent of UK women ages eighteen to twenty-four, for instance, have been sexually harassed in public places.[31] And verbal harassment, like assault, has been linked to physical and mental health conditions like depression and insomnia.[32] This means the majority of women – I'd venture to say nearly all – have faced enough sexual violations to impact their physical and/or mental health.

That's not counting all the other types of sexism that take a toll on victims' well-being. Depression is three times as common in women who have faced sex-based discrimination, and women who make less money than their male counterparts are more prone to depression and anxiety.[33] Similarly, trans women who have experienced discrimination are more susceptible to PTSD and suicidal thoughts.[34] As Josefina can attest, other axes of identity like social class also increase vulnerability to trauma. Those of lower socioeconomic status are more prone to sexual abuse, according to studies in Iceland and the US.[35] And women of color are not just frequently targeted but also mistreated by the criminal justice system and viewed through the lens of stereotypes that render them hyper-sexual or submissive.[36]

When all these forms of oppression converge, many marginalized people end up enduring a series of traumas for a prolonged time period. This can lead to complex PTSD, a disorder characterized by hard-to-control emotions, difficulty sustaining relationships, and a persistent sense of shame on top of typical PTSD symptoms. Complex PTSD has been acknowledged by psychiatrists, supported by brain imaging studies, and discussed in scientific journals for over three decades. The World Health Organization includes it in its diagnostic guide, the International Classification of Diseases. Yet it hasn't made it into the Diagnostic and Statistical Manual used by American mental health professionals, which means trauma symptoms fail to be attributed to the events behind them.[37]

Some diagnoses women disproportionately receive may often be misdiagnosed complex PTSD, or otherwise stem from trauma. Take borderline personality disorder (BPD), defined by volatile moods, unstable self-image, and dramatic relationships. Its association with the "crazy woman" stereotype positions it among the most stigmatized mental illnesses, and it is almost always linked to trauma. In one Brown University study, 81% of BPD patients had experienced childhood abuse, and 90% had faced neglect.[38] Psychologist Diane Gehart tells me BPD would be better classified as a trauma disorder than a personality disorder. A personality disorder diagnosis can feel like a life sentence, as it implies the mental illness is who you are. Survivors feel as if something's amiss in their wiring when they're having a warranted response to trauma. But whether someone has true BPD or misdiagnosed complex PTSD, such trauma-based pathologies are not set in stone. Many people stop meeting the criteria for BPD after receiving therapies like dialectical behavior therapy or psychoanalysis.[39] Yet the inferiority complex someone acquires through mental health stigma may last. When someone's trauma remains unacknowledged and they're told they're naturally anxious, depressed, or unwell, they may feel helpless and ashamed. The pattern repeats itself with many conditions: Society makes women and sex and gender-diverse people mentally ill, then demeans them for their illness as if the issue is with their brain chemistry.

Psychologists believe BPD stems from growing up in an environment where you're gaslit and dismissed. Where your feelings are minimized. This is known as an invalidating environment.[40] I can't think of a more invalidating environment for women than today's patriarchy. There's a reason "believe women" is a popular feminist outcry: Women are habitually invalidated. Society silences and second-guesses them. Anyone exposed to this environment every day would struggle with mental health.

The Female Body, Shaped by Trauma

Many things that appear wrong with women's bodies, as with their minds, stem from trauma incurred through their upbringing and culture's wrongs. The number of adverse childhood experiences someone has faced predicts their chances of developing illnesses like cancer, diabetes, and cardiovascular disease.[41] And women who have survived sexual trauma are more likely to deal with chronic pain.[42] Even "typical" issues like period problems can be traced back to the disconcerting prevalence of trauma. Physical, emotional, and sexual abuse are linked to menstrual pain, PMS, PMDD, and difficult menopause symptoms.[43] How could something so invisible, so insidious, have such a lasting, tangible impact on our bodies and brains? One straightforward explanation is that trauma and shame stop us from caring for ourselves. Sexual trauma survivors, for instance, are less likely to attend cervical cancer screenings because they're triggering.[44] In addition, traumatic events contribute to physical illness via mental illness. Depression is a risk factor for chronic pain conditions like fibromyalgia, rheumatoid arthritis, and migraines.[45] And so trauma creates a debilitating cycle of pain: It makes women depressed, increasing their risk for chronic pain – which often makes them more depressed.

Trauma may also directly alter a survivor's physiology. As psychiatrist Bessel van der Kolk notes in *The Body Keeps the Score*, trauma can induce a chronic stress response. Healthy levels of the stress hormone cortisol are important for immune regulation. So, chronic stress can lead to immune dysregulation. The survivor's immune system, like their brain, may become hyper-responsive to perceived threats. In this state of overdrive, it can attack the body's own tissue – the basis of autoimmune illnesses.[46] A study of over 100,000 people found that autoimmune disorders like Crohn's disease, celiac disease, multiple sclerosis, and psoriasis were 46% more prevalent in PTSD patients.[47] Perhaps one reason autoimmune diseases are twice as common in women is that PTSD is as well.[48] Chronic stress like that incurred through harmful sexual experiences can even affect brain development. In one Rutgers study, female rats placed in cages with sexually aggressive older males during puberty later had difficulty learning and did not care for their offspring. And the new cells their brains generated were dying at an alarming rate.[49] Other research has shown that stress affects brain cell production in other mammals including humans – another way sexual trauma can compromise women's physical and mental health.[50]

When I look at my own body in the mirror, I see many pathways from trauma to pain, all intersecting, intertwining, and diverging. Some are lightly paved while others are so worn, they feel like parts of me. I see a jaw that was clenching with anger from having my voice silenced. A clenching that spread all the way down to my pelvis, creating tension.[51] I see eyes that were always on the lookout in a world where the streets are unsafe for women. A nervous system on high alert, waking me up to nondescript dangers at night. I see a body that was ogled at and commented on before I learned how to honor and safeguard it. I see a gut disrupted by disordered eating, a method to protect from this attention. I see a stomach constantly sucked in, trying to shrink myself, making it hard to breathe in and out. I see a back and shoulders strung out from the stress of bending over my laptop, hiding behind Adam's curse, working my worries away. I see a body and mind that have spent their lives on guard from men who took my "no" as a "try harder," from eyes that lingered lower than they should, from sexist assumptions at the tips of people's tongues. My awareness split, with half on my somatic sensations and half monitoring the scene for safety threats. I was too far outside myself to notice discomfort until it became unbearable. So it lingered, passing for normalcy. This was part of being a woman, after all.

Being "crazy," having issues in the bedroom, struggling with pain – these are deemed defining traits of femininity. They are mocked and scorned. But when we do this, we are looking down upon trauma survivors. An examination of trauma's impact reveals that physical, mental, and sexual suffering are not endemic to womanhood. They are endemic to a culture where women are constantly fielding attacks on their safety. Rather than deem women's physical and mental maladies evidence of their inadequacy or ridiculousness, we must have compassion for those who have endured the experiences underlying these challenges. We must admire the strength it takes to routinely surmount trauma, even as your mind and body take a hit. Even – no, especially – as you are accused of being the hitter.

Chapter 9

Sexy But Not Sexual

Do you remember Abby from our first chapter? She spent years pleading for doctors to take the pain that plagued her sex life seriously – until in one last-ditch effort, she started bringing her boyfriend to appointments. Once he attested that she couldn't have sex, doctors suddenly began listening. Her other strategy to muster up concern for her reproductive health was hiding that she didn't want kids. "The fact that I was in excruciating pain and couldn't eat and couldn't enjoy sex wasn't enough," she says.

Today, the Victorian myth of female passionlessness exists side by side with rape culture. Women are expected to be sexual objects but not seek out sex. To look desirable but lack desire. To be wanted but not want. To be, as Paris Hilton described herself to *Rolling Stone* in 2003, "sexy but not sexual."[1] Hilton elaborated to *Vanity Fair*: "I think I'm sexual in pictures and the way I dress ... but at home I'm really not like that."[2] The seductive image she projected to the world was just that: an image. Which is what women's sexuality itself has been flattened to. At the time these words were spoken, Hollywood and magazines idealized underweight young women. Passively posed yet revealingly dressed, erotically immature yet consumable. Hairless vulvas came into vogue, perpetuating an image of simultaneous sexual lackingness and accessibility.[3] Labiaplasty and breast implants were on the rise, helping women meet beauty standards while risking reduction of sensation.[4] Women's ability to perform sexiness was prized over their own sexuality. It still is. And this has devastating effects on our sex lives and our health.

"Any Hole Will Do"

In 2012, hundreds of Australian women pressed charges against pharmaceutical company Johnson & Johnson. The corporation's mesh implants – devices surgically inserted into the pelvis to treat weak or damaged tissue – made sex painful for them. In emails leaked during the 2017 trial, a company gynecologist argued: "Sodomy could be a good alternative!" Women's orifices were interchangeable as long as at least one was available to men. One victim told *The Guardian*: "The suggestion that women who are unable to have vaginal intercourse should practice anal instead completely devalues a woman's right to a full and healthy sex life as an active, empowered, and fulfilled participant. It suggests that a woman is nothing more than a receptacle to satisfy men and that 'any hole will do.'"[5]

The conception of women as sexy, not sexual, means women's ability to please men is prioritized over their own pleasure – not just in the bedroom but in the doctor's office. And when someone you trust to improve your well-being ignores or hurts your sexual well-being, this is a devastating betrayal. Reports have recently emerged of loop electrosurgical excision procedures (LEEPs), where a heated wire removes precancerous cells in the cervix, reducing sexual pleasure. In one 1,600-woman survey, a third of patients experienced pain during or after sex following their LEEPs. For 41% of those with this side effect, it was still happening after a year or more.[6] In another study, women reported lower sexual and orgasmic satisfaction seven months post-LEEP than pre-LEEP.[7] Some patients even lose the ability to orgasm. These effects are not typically anticipated due to ignorance of the cervical nerves and their role in sexual response.[8] Half a million LEEPs take place in the US alone every year.[9]

Kate Orson was referred to a clinic in Glasgow, Scotland for a LEEP in 2003 after two pap smears detected abnormal cervical cells. Not only did her stomach muscles get so weak it became hard to sit, but she lost her libido, sex became painful, and she could not orgasm. Her pelvic muscles would contract as if she were orgasming, but she felt nothing. She saw another doctor, who said she must have "a little bit of scarring" and suggested burning off the scar tissue. "How can you solve the problem with something that sounds really similar to what caused the problem?" she remembers thinking. "I just didn't go back at all because I thought, how are they going to help me?" Kate now runs a Facebook group for women dealing with side effects from LEEPs, and she commonly hears stories of doctors denying the problem, lacking solutions, or claiming the issue's unrelated to the LEEP. "Doctors won't acknowledge the side effects because unlike male pelvic organs, female organs have not been properly researched," she explains. "So there's very little awareness that the cervix is involved in pleasure. Even pain in the cervix is not recognized by some doctors."

The side effects LEEP patients experience make sense from an anatomical perspective. Three pairs of nerves carry pleasure signals from the cervix to the brain, which is why removal of the cervix often compromises orgasmic ability.[10] Yet the uterus is seen as a reproductive vehicle for men or children to utilize, not something for women themselves to enjoy. It's how society sees the female body as a whole. Women's bodies are not seen as sexually functional apparatuses, so their pleasure is not considered in their care. "Doctors, especially the older ones, were taught in medical school that the cervix has no nerve endings, which isn't true," says Kate. Her LEEP affected areas of her life she was not expecting:

> I would watch a TV program, and people having sex would just look like aliens to me, because I think the cervix is the center of our being as sexual human beings. So, if you traumatize that and cut it and damage it, you don't even feel like a human being anymore. I've never felt in such a weird mental state. It's not even depression, because you've just had your being cut from you. It's very bizarre.

Kate has regained functioning over time as her nerve endings have had the chance to regrow. But not everyone in her Facebook group has been so lucky. "Some are harmed forever, and it just really traumatized them," she says. "They can't have a relationship ever again." How could we allow this? By seeing women as sexy, not sexual. Doctors, like the rest of the world, fail to realize our pleasure – not our presentation or performance – is core to who we are.

"Just Get on the Pill"

Many women may have never heard of LEEPs or pelvic mesh implants. But at least 500 million women worldwide have taken something else: hormonal birth control.[11] From 2006 to 2010, 88% of sexually experienced American women had used the birth control pill, patch, injection, ring, or intrauterine device (IUD).[12] And even these widely used contraceptives can lead to decreased sex drive, painful sex, diminished clitoral size and blood flow, and low free testosterone, which can thin out vulvar tissue and cause discomfort.[13] One 2016 study found that after three months on oral contraceptives, women had lower testosterone levels and reported less desire, arousal, and pleasure than those on a placebo.[14] In another 900-woman study, those on low-dose estrogen contraceptive pills reported more pelvic pain, including twice the incidence of pain during or after climax, compared to those not on the pill.[15] Yet another study of 1,100 women found those on hormonal birth control had more arousal, orgasm, and lubrication difficulties than those using non-hormonal methods.[16] Even the copper IUD, a non-hormonal device recommended to avoid these issues, can lead to heavy, long, painful periods.[17] Perhaps this doesn't sound alarming if you've been taught period pain is part of being female. Perhaps none of these side effects feel like a big deal if you've learned your role in sex is to provide enjoyment, not enjoy yourself.

All drugs have side effects, and many don't experience these ones. Some see no changes or even improvements in sexual functioning or menstrual symptoms after starting contraceptives.[18] But the lack of awareness or better options speaks to the valuing of women's sexual availability to men over their own satisfaction. Women are expected by default to bear the burden of birth control, as Krystale E. Littlejohn illustrates in *Just Get on the Pill*.[19] Meanwhile, many men complain that condoms or withdrawal detract too much from their satisfaction. Women's pain and pleasurelessness come second to their male partners' slightly diminished pleasure. Even the progressive Planned Parenthood warns in an eerily rapey informational page that withdrawal is "hard" because "you have to pull out right around the time those pleasurable sex feelings are the most intense, which many people aren't willing to do when it comes down to it."[20] Never mind that some women stay on birth control when it prevents them from enjoying "pleasurable sex feelings" at all. Men are deemed entitled to pleasure even when it puts their partners at risk and violates their consent. Yet women must fight to have their pleasure and pain taken into consideration.

Some women go on birth control at young ages and don't realize their problems stem from it.[21] After all, many of the side effects – painful periods, painful sex, difficulty with arousal and orgasm – are considered normal. And so we have another self-perpetuating cycle: When women don't get help for these issues, they become very common and appear, indeed, intrinsic to womanhood. Women in the US are also twice as likely as men to be prescribed antidepressants, which can cause low libido and anorgasmia.[22] Because these side effects are under-researched and infrequently discussed, women like me and Margaret don't always learn about them until they experience them – only to have them brushed off, once again, as part of being female. The overuse of medical interventions that diminish women's pleasure and increase their pain could partially explain many "natural" gender differences like the orgasm gap, women's supposedly lower sex drives, and the prevalence of female sexual pain.

Not Sexy Enough to Be Sexual

Women's sex lives suffer when they learn they are designed to provide pleasure but not obtain it. In a 2011 University of Michigan study involving interviews with eighty-five college students, women believed their partners' satisfaction marked the success of a hookup. "I will do everything in my power to, like whoever I'm with, to get them off," one said. "It makes me feel like I'm good at sex … because in a hookup, that's really all you have." Another woman stated: "I don't feel like I've had a sexual experience if the guy doesn't come."[23] It's as if the pleasure women offer men is a proxy for their own. It's as if their sexiness is the entirety of their sexuality. Kaytlin remembers feeling so much pressure to give partners orgasms, she couldn't focus on her own. Or as Sophie puts it:

I was kind of trying to put on an act, especially in the beginning. I was like, "Ooh, how am I supposed to look? Am I doing this right?" I was being very performance-oriented: "If I do this, I'm gonna look good" or "this is how I'm supposed to do it," instead of being in tune with how my body actually wanted to move. I never watched a lot of porn, but I'm sure that was a factor. And not really ever seeing an example of what female sexuality could look like in its full expression.

Mainstream porn and other media teach us men's pleasure is the goal of sex, while women's is a bonus – often to further please men. A 2018 analysis of Pornhub's fifty all-time most popular videos found that only 18% of women – compared to 78% of men – were depicted as reaching climax. The most common activities eliciting these orgasms (if we generously assume they were real orgasms) were vaginal and anal intercourse, not acts geared specifically toward female pleasure.[24] The goal was not to show how women achieve climax but to display sexy moans, movements, and faces. In contrast, porn videos – even many made "for women" – overwhelmingly culminate with "money shots" where men get off.

The depiction of women as pleasure providers, not seekers, keeps them self-monitoring during sex – a recipe for pleasurelessness. Thirty-two percent of women in one *Cosmo* survey said that when they didn't orgasm, it was because they were in their heads or focused on their looks.[25] Insidiously, it's often body parts with high pleasure potential that end up objects of women's scrutiny. "Some part of me still viewed my pussy as deformed or broken based on the molestation experience I had," says Josefina. "I felt uncomfortable, especially if someone was going to see me or go down on me. The perception I had was that I was ugly and broken when it came to my genitals specifically, and that contributed to me feeling unworthy as a woman." Sophie would shut down when partners tried to please her due to similar insecurities. "I felt my pussy was weird," she shares. "I was already judging how I felt and how my body was responding or not. I always thought I needed to lose weight and was hyper-critical. I was embarrassed to really be seen. I was like, 'How do I look? Does my body look weird?' I didn't really see my pussy as beautiful." In a world where we valued women's sexuality over their sexiness, we wouldn't need to see our bodies as beautiful to enjoy sex. We could simply live in them, without evaluating ourselves from the outside. If only it were so simple.

Sexuality Beyond Cultural Prescriptions of Sexiness

With women's bodies prized for how they look above what they do, we end up hating on our bodies when we could be celebrating accomplishments like childbirth. Sixty-nine percent of women are dissatisfied with their postpartum figures.[26] "Giving birth definitely changed the way my body looks, and so it's been a journey," says Ayelet. "At the beginning after giving birth, I'd look in the mirror and go back and forth between these thought processes of 'ugh, my body just doesn't look the way it used to look; that's sad' but also to this other extreme: 'But yeah, hold on – you literally just birthed a human through your body.'" The pressure to self-monitor also hits older women hard. When women ages forty to sixty-nine are asked what would improve their sexual satisfaction, the most common response is body confidence.[27] They don't feel sexy enough to be sexual. And since women are supposedly unsexy after a certain age, their sexuality comes to seem less important. Older women's doctors don't always ask about their sexual functioning even though sexual dysfunction can point toward conditions like heart disease, infections, cancer, and diabetes that then get missed.[28] This perpetuates the myth that older women are, by nature, not just sexless but sick. It makes their pleasurelessness and pain yet another self-fulfilling prophecy.

People experience a general "ick factor" around older people's sexuality, says Joan Price, the sex educator quoted in chapter 3. But it's women in particular who are deemed irrelevant once they outgrow cultural prescriptions for sexiness. "We see it in advertising: Even something that is marketed to older people has younger models," says Joan. "We're not seen, we're not heard; we're either invisible or we're put down." Yet the reality of older women's sex lives squashes the misconception that women must fit narrow beauty standards to enjoy their bodies. Older women often report improved intimacy due to increased confidence, self-knowledge, and connection with partners.[29] As Joan puts it:

> We have a lot of experience. We know what we like. We know better how to communicate that to a partner. We've made our mistakes. If we are lucky, now we know how to stop making them. It is not automatic; we have to decide this is a value for us to advocate for our own pleasure. And to be able to take it all with a sense of humor. We certainly find life funnier as we age, and the more we can bring laughter into our bedroom, the more we are going to enjoy being in that bedroom. We learn to celebrate what we've got because our bodies are capable of great pleasure – great sensual and sexual pleasure lifelong.

Women's sexuality continues to expand and thrive long past the point when they're supposed to lose their sexiness. Women's physicality continues to bring them joy from the inside no matter what others say about the outside. Women continue to find blessings in their bodies irrespective of the curses they supposedly carry. More blessings than are visible to the eye.

Part II

Paradise Gained

"Why do women have to go through this?" Leia whimpered from a white bed, immobilized from the waist down by an epidural that blunted but did not block her labor contractions.

"Because Eve ate that apple, remember?" her husband RJ replied.

I'd been in this dimly lit hospital basement room since 4 a.m. massaging Leia, repositioning her, and guiding her to breathe deeply as her birth doula. We were heading into the afternoon now. At this moment, I walked from a small armchair in the corner toward the bed.

"I've been thinking about that," I told RJ. "If God really put a curse on Eve, what if that curse wasn't meant to be permanent? What if it were something he knew Eve could unwind?"

"What do you mean?"

"Well, what if it were an interesting challenge to figure out how to break the curse? Our lives would be boring if we'd just stayed in the Garden of Eden."

"Does that mean this can be a pleasant experience?" Leia asked between groans.

"I don't know," I replied. "Maybe not right here, right now. But I wonder if, one day, we could live in a world where it is."

Chapter 10

Womanhood Is Not an Illness

In 2018, I grew ill, and no one could tell me what ailed me. A series of symptoms including chronic headaches, heart palpitations, and the aforementioned bladder pain took over my life. Doctors offered me such speculations as "you seem anxious," "you're traveling too much," and "you just need to stop eating dairy." The solutions they proposed, mostly antidepressants and other medications, made me worse. So I turned to holistic healers, who had similarly dismissive theories: I had "emotions stuck in my body." I'd "manifested" my illness. The problem was "energetic." It was the same covert misogyny dressed in spiritual language. From mainstream and alternative providers alike, I received the familiar suggestion that perhaps my body was designed to suffer. "Is it really that bad if your neck cracks? It doesn't interfere with your functioning, does it?" "It probably hurts when you get aroused because of the position you're masturbating in." "You'll realize if you pay attention that it's your period bringing on the insomnia." "You can expect joint issues as you get older; it's wear and tear." I was twenty-eight.

Then a friend introduced me to Sarah Ramey, author of *The Lady's Handbook for Her Mysterious Illness*, whose story of medical mistreatment makes mine look like a breeze. She has a word for women like me and her: "WOMIs" or "women with mysterious illnesses." Sarah warned me about doctors who deem women's symptoms psychological and suggested I look into functional medicine, which treats many maladies mainstream providers brush off. Finally, I found a doctor who diagnosed me with chronic Lyme disease. After working with her for a few months, I began waking up glad to see the sun outside my window rather than dreading another day in my body.

It's Not Normal

Thanks to the view of femaleness itself as an illness, women like me have had to fight for diagnoses and treatments. Many knew all along that their pain was not normal, but the hard part was getting others to believe them. When doctor after doctor said Abby's endometriosis was untreatable – or not bad enough to warrant treatment – she started reading medical journals and showing providers articles. "Beyond the research and nagging, I think it was my persistent insistence that there was a problem," she says. Other women were resigned to their pain until they found clinicians who questioned it. Celia recalls:

> My current gynecologist is wonderful, and finally, I told her about painful sex. And when I said, "Oh well yeah, it's always been like this, it's not new," she looked at me and said, "I'm gonna try something." And she did that pelvic exam thing where it feels like she's crushing your ovaries – or at least that's how it always felt to me – and it hurt so bad. And I looked at her and I said: "Is that supposed to hurt?" She said, "No, no, that's not supposed to hurt." And mind you, *it's always hurt*. I just never said anything.

America's turning point also came when she found a doctor who took her suffering seriously. As I discussed in chapter 2, most doctors don't use highly sensitive tests for urinary tract infections, since they're among the many under-researched women's health issues. However, more and more providers are adopting newer testing methods.[1] A few years ago, America connected with a urologist who looks for UTIs by examining urine under a microscope. "He has been able to find the exact bacteria present in my bladder and what antibiotics it is and is not resistant to," she says. "Based on the protocol that I have been on since 2020, I can now say I am 90% symptom-free and don't have to take antibiotics on a daily basis anymore. I lived with a ten-year infection, and the pain was unimaginable. Since 2023, I no longer feel my bladder. Before, it was always present. Burning and on fire 100% of the time. Not anymore."

My journey with bladder pain was similar. Along with my functional medicine doctor, I found a urologist who identified the bacteria in my urinary tract using a testing method called liquid broth culture. Lo and behold – despite my supposedly incurable illness – antibiotics got me almost completely better too. The last lingering symptoms went away after treating Lyme and coinfections, which can lurk in the bladder and trap other bacteria there, leading to UTIs.[2] After describing myself as a "former IC patient" in an interstitial cystitis Facebook group a few months later, I received angry comments demanding I revise my post to avoid implying IC can be overcome. Many see such stories as giving false hope. That's how stubborn the notion of women's cursedness is. While every patient is different, many cases of chronic bladder pain have identifiable, curable causes.[3] Medicine and science have just not, up to this point, looked for them. Doctors' unawareness of what causes women's pain doesn't mean we were just born with it – or that we have to die with it.

WOMIs Supporting WOMIs

I am where I am today because of Sarah and other WOMIs I've met along the way. In a world that's not set up to support women's wellness, pleasure, or comfort, we've had to advocate for one another. For her part, Abby wrote her memoir *Ask Me About My Uterus* so people grow aware of conditions like endometriosis and stop dismissing their discomfort. "I was raised to do everything in my power to make sure people didn't know I was on my period," she explains. "For years, I had bad periods. For years, I had weird symptoms. I never paid attention, but if I had, who would I have told? There's this idea that you need to preserve the feminine mystique. That serves men because men don't want it to be ruined for them." She hopes others in this position will come across her book and finally find answers. "What haunts me are the women in my mother's demographic who have been enduring excruciating sex and raising their kids and holding down jobs and trying to mitigate their pain without anybody knowing about it, and they've been doing it for thirty years," she says. "I like the idea that this book is going to be in libraries and find places I can't get to. In those moments where they're exhausted, where they can't tell anyone, it's nice to feel like I've offered something."

Tara also now offers others the fruits of her healing journey. But first, she had to take her health into her own hands. Vulvodynia, like many women's health conditions, doesn't have a standard treatment, but Tara had an idea.[4] Her mother had used magnets to treat nerve pain from fibromyalgia, and since Tara suspected her vulvodynia stemmed from nerve pain, she tried putting a magnet into a dilator – a tube-shaped device that goes in the vagina. She inserted the dilator half an hour before sex, and by the end, she was crying – not from pain, but from happiness. It was the first time in five years that she'd had sex with her husband comfortably. Through her company VuvaTech, she now sells magnetic dilators like the one that helped her. She tirelessly works to get the word out, as many still don't know about vulvodynia:

> I'll talk to a seventy-year-old woman and they'll be like, "I never told my doctor I have pain." Women are embarrassed about it. They don't want to talk about it, and therefore, no one's really pushed their physician to figure it out. So they've gotten told things like "just relax" or "take an antidepressant." People listen to their doctors way too much like they are the Bible. They're like, "I need to ask a doctor before I use a dilator." I'm like, "Why do you have to ask a sixty-five-year-old man?" It's ingrained. You don't have to ask your doctor to take care of yourself. Some people have diabetes, and some people have to take insulin every day. We have vulvodynia, and we have to use a dilator. And until they can figure out what will make vulvodynia go away, it's what we have to do. But at least there's something.

This Type of Body

"I don't feel like we're meant to suffer; I don't understand why so many of us have to," muses Tara. "I'm a go-getter; I'm not a 'poor me' person. I'm more of an 'I have to figure out how to fix this' type of person." So, she's spent the past few years speaking to physicians, physical therapists, and patients about vulvodynia. And over time, she's observed a pattern: Many patients have what she calls "this type of body." They have co-occurring problems like hypermobility, chemical sensitivities, gut issues like small intestinal bacterial overgrowth, and intolerance to foods and drinks that contain chemicals called histamines. "They all have this laundry list of the same issues," she explains. "If you ask people who have vulvodynia, they'll tell you they have nerve pain or fibromyalgia. Something is just off, and our nervous systems are on high alert."

Some vulvodynia patients have told Tara their host of problems was brought on by antibiotics, which can kill helpful bacteria, creating imbalances in the gut microbiome. This in turn can lead to histamine intolerance, a condition causing allergy-like reactions to histamines. There has, in fact, been research linking histamine intolerance to vulvodynia, along with other forms of pelvic pain like IC.[5] Histamines are hard to avoid, as they exist in the body along with certain foods and beverages. The histamines in the body can be released in response to EMFs – electromagnetic fields emitted by cell phones, computers, and WiFi routers – as well as excess estrogen stemming from hormone-disrupting chemicals.[6] "I ask people, 'Can you drink wine?' And they say, 'No, I take one sip and I feel it through my body,'" says Tara. "Red wine is one of the highest histamine foods you can put in your body."[7] She believes many cases of vulvodynia stem from histamine intolerance, which in turn stems from dysbiosis – an imbalance of helpful and harmful gut bacteria. Many everyday elements of the modern world including environmental toxins, processed foods, stress, antibiotics, and other medications cause dysbiosis.[8]

When Tara described this pattern to me, I had déjà vu. It reminded me of Sarah's theory of WOMIs. Her book postulates that women with mysterious illnesses are reacting to harmful aspects of modern life we ignore: antibiotic overuse, poor nutrition, hormone-disruptive chemicals, high-stress lifestyles, inadequate rest, social disconnection. These factors can lead to dysbiosis as well as dysfunction of the hypothalamic–pituitary–adrenal (HPA) axis, which throws off the stress response and contributes to neurological disorders.[9] They're some of the same factors I've cited as contributors to period pain and PMS. Sarah believes even women with "normal" issues like these are a type of WOMI. Whether we're struggling with autoimmune diseases, chronic pain, or hormonal imbalances, many of us have "this type of body" – one that's reactive to its environment. We're all reacting to similar issues. And the core issue behind them is society not prioritizing people's well-being – especially women's. It's why we've turned a blind eye to these issues all along. As Sarah puts it:

> Women's problems don't get studied, and so doctors don't have the tools to remedy those problems. And because they can't remedy the problems, that makes the doctors feel uncomfortable. So instead of saying "I don't know what to do here," they say, "This is not a problem in the first place." Because saying "I don't know" is never an option, but saying "I don't believe you" almost always is. And this has major consequences beyond getting your feelings hurt. When a doctor normalizes or dismisses or diminishes the patient and says, "Your mountain is actually a molehill," this is like having your house burn down, and then you call the fire department and they say, "Oh sweetie, all houses burn down" or "I actually don't believe that your house is burning down – we're not coming." And then the house burns down, and the result is catastrophic. You, the caller, can't force them to put out the fire. You can't force them to help you. They've decided that it's normal for female houses to burn down, and so that is exactly what happens.

And as WOMIs' houses burn down, many other houses are burning down too. Maybe more slowly, maybe less noticeably, but we're all affected by society's neglect for women's well-being. We're all affected by our culture of high stress, lack of community, overworking, unhealthy relationships with food, oppression leading to inadequate care, and medicine that offers quick fixes without addressing root causes. For now, it's primarily women who are saying, "There's a fire!" But if we don't start believing women – taking their health concerns seriously, learning what causes them, studying how to solve them – everyone else will burn down with us.

Illness Isn't Punishment

It took me years to unpack the assumption that my pain was not only normal but just. As I saw others out and about enjoying life while I silently suffered, I couldn't help but feel less fortunate, less favored. I must have been despised by whatever force designed me inferiorly. It was hard to accept that perhaps bad things do happen to good people. Though I was never told this outright, it was ingrained in me that people get what they deserve. These feelings escalated when, after a couple years of reprieve, I faced a major relapse in 2021. I was a WOMI, a woman with this type of body, and my list of inter-related issues piled up: Lyme, mold toxicity, vaginal infections, strange tingling sensations. Immersed in the new age community, I heard the same things: I was "manifesting disease." I had to take "radical self-responsibility" and see I had a hand in this. Friends and healers all had different stories about why I'd called it in: Because I wasn't open to finding love. Because I was too focused on love. Because I was deficient in feminine energy. Because I wasn't meditating daily. Because I didn't fully believe I would get better. Because I was too attached to getting better. They might as well have told me this was happening because Eve ate that apple. It was the same logic: My discomfort was paying a cosmic debt. I'd messed up in God knows what way, and now, I was getting what I asked for.

At the time, I lacked the strength to challenge these ideas. I scrambled to change my ways so as not to call in sickness. I meditated twice a day. I did flowy dances to be "in my feminine." I burned a bunch of things associated with an old flame after someone claimed my "attachment" to him was the issue. I tried every diet out there. And I grew more ill, exhausted, and self-loathing. Surprisingly, it was a conversation with a Christian friend that introduced me to another way of thinking. She was describing a past miscarriage and how it connected to her faith. "I don't think my miscarriage was God's doing," she said. "I think God allowed darkness to exist because that gives life more meaning. But he doesn't want to see us unhappy. So when we are, he finds a way to turn that darkness into light." She evoked the analogy of a painting: Even if our lives are full of shadowy images, God can take a paintbrush and blend the colors until the picture portrays something beautiful. As she spoke about her adopted son, I understood what she meant. I began to comprehend a different higher power than the one who had cursed me. One that believed we need not suffer for our supposed sins.

I wasn't raised with religious shame or dogma. I grew up attending a liberal Jewish temple that taught us not to take the Torah literally, and a Quaker meeting house where services were more like informal discussions. Yet the punishing God had seeped into my consciousness, as fire-and-brimstone views of pain as punishment extend beyond religion. They stem from ancient Greek philosophers who looked down upon women and the flesh. They stem from church figures like St. Augustine and Jerome much more than Christ himself.[10] They show up in new age notions of manifesting illness. They show up in so many people's nagging sense that they must have done something to cause their struggles. It's time we break free from this philosophy and theology that haunt us regardless of our creed. It's time we unconditionally advocate for our access to compassionate care. It's time we support others to find the same, not blame or shame them for their supposedly broken bodies. It's time we see our bodies as whole. Holy. Wholly undeserving of disease.

At last, I stopped trying to fix the imagined flaws that allegedly made me sick and sought real recovery. If any component of my psyche was making me ill, it was the belief that I'd attracted illness. I did not have to correct my imperfections to receive mercy. I had to show myself mercy. To be gentle with my body. To find people who understood what really ailed me, commit myself to treatments that worked, and allow myself time to play and rest. That was it. The female illness epidemic is much bigger than women. The belief in Eve's curse is a belief in Adam's and humankind's. It's a belief that we have erred for existing in our bodies. That's why, in leading pleasurable lives, women can pave a new path for humanity. A path to a place where we see we deserve not punishment but praise, reward, and healing. No matter who we are or what we've done. There's always a way to smudge the colors in the painting until something bright emerges. Whatever God we do or don't believe in, we can be that forgiving force for ourselves.

Chapter 11

Period Pleasure

Since we've traversed dark times together, I'll tell you a lighter tale. The other night, I was lying in bed reminiscing on a past dalliance when I had a novel experience: I orgasmed in response to nothing but that fantasy. Touch-free orgasm is a known phenomenon, but it had not come to me so effortlessly before.[1] Sure enough, I woke up the next morning with bloody sheets. The kind that signify pleasure, not pain. I was headed into my wettest week: the five or so days when erotic sensations heighten and my body basically drips lube. I've discovered several new sexual capabilities during menstruation before learning to experience them all month long. I used to think I could only have one orgasm at a time until I started experiencing multiple orgasms during my period. When my body is unusually responsive, I can sense it's around the corner. I anticipate it with interest, not apprehension. This is not my cursed week, my alone week, my wrapped up in a ball week. I call it my wet week.

Lots of people acknowledge period pain but not period pleasure. In fact, I fear your eyes will roll at this phrase. But this is not a tampon commercial about how you can push through pain and be a boss babe all month long. It's an exploration of what menstruation might look like outside patriarchal views of it as a curse. It'd look different for everyone, but I know this: There would be more pleasure and less pain.

Periods Are Painful ... Yay?

In 2018, the internet celebrated a statement by University College London professor John Guillebaud to the publication *Quartz*: Period pain, he said, can be "almost as bad as a heart attack." At last, women's suffering was acknowledged. Guillebaud's words were praised by publications from *Cosmo* to *Marie Claire*, which declared, "Doctors have finally ruled menstrual cramps are as painful as heart attacks. We could have told you that." We, presumably, being women.[2] But was this proclamation such a victory? *Elle* called it an "improvement on the previous medical advice that recommended ibuprofen as 'good enough' to prescribe."[3] Yet ibuprofen generally *is* enough – if it's needed at all – unless someone is sick. If a patient has such severe menstrual pain that over-the-counter meds won't resolve it, endocrinologist Aimee Eyvazzadeh is "very concerned," she says. "I'm very suspicious for fibroids, endometriosis, adenomyosis, or ovarian cysts." Articles implying most women relate to heart-attack-level pain depict it as non-pathological, stopping menstruators from investigating their discomfort's origins. In more recent viral YouTube videos, men learn "what it feels like to have a period" via pain-simulating machines that make them shout in agony, encouraging empathy for those with bad periods while normalizing them at the same time.[4]

Many see it as a win when women's pain is validated, but validation is not enough. Prizing women for the pain they endure risks further defining women by pain. Women need to be heard, but it can't stop there. We must empathize with women's pain but see that it is not what we were made for.

It is not what it means to be a woman. And that's why we need to talk about positive menstrual experiences. Pain is not the only sensation a uterus can spawn, nor should it be a common one even if it is today. Discomfort is not universal, and desired changes like rises in creativity, mental agility, and body attunement are common too.[5] Negative views of periods make girls dread puberty and adulthood, and this dread does no good. It either provokes worry over something that turns out fine or makes what is already bad worse. Instead of validating women's pain alone, let's validate their pleasure. Instead of hammering home that periods are awful for many in the present, let's look toward a better future.

Breaking the Curse

Lauren Schulte Wang used to dread her periods. They were so heavy and painful, she had to stop what she was doing and lie down. She became bloated while she bled, and afterward, she got yeast infections almost every month. "I simply accepted that uncomfortable periods were my plight in life," she recalls. "My mom and Oma (maternal grandmother) had very heavy and painful periods to the point that they would vomit from the pain. I never vomited from pain, but that's to say they taught me that my symptoms were more or less normal. I never expected that my period could or should be anything other than uncomfortable. I did not believe that I should expect better. I hear the same refrain from many people today. It's so ingrained in us from a young age that periods suck, we don't even realize they suck anymore."

But after a few years, Lauren noticed something. "I remember in high school teaching all of my friends when they had bad cramps to take their tampons out, and they agreed that it helped," she says. She started researching tampons and learned they could disrupt vaginal pH levels, trap harmful bacteria in the vagina, and absorb good bacteria.[6] "I also started researching how and where tampons were manufactured, only to discover that they're all made from the same handful of manufacturers but sold under different brands. I was pretty ticked off because I'd wasted so much money trying different brands of tampons that were all the same," Lauren says. "If tampons were invented today, they'd never pass approval from the FDA. We wouldn't walk around with a piece of cotton in our mouths all day; our mouths are full of bacteria. And I think that wearing tampons inside of the vagina is as silly as that concept." Concerning levels of heavy metals have also been found in tampons, though some research has found no correlation between tampon use and period pain.[7] The jury's out on how common it is to experience menstrual issues from tampons, but Lauren could tell she did. Menstrual cups were more body-safe but still uncomfortable for her, so she started her own menstrual disc company FLEX. Since switching her supplies, she no longer gets period cramps or yeast infections. "I have gotten my period on my wedding day, at all six Burning Man events that I have attended, and seemingly every other important life milestone," she says.

Getting rid of period pain is not always as simple as swapping out products, but other women have accomplished it. The same things that helped with Meg's PMS – more down time, less caffeine, honoring her emotions, asserting boundaries, eating in line with her changing needs throughout her cycle – also helped eliminate her cramps and breakouts. Now, she feels a sense of calm and self-attunement during menstruation. "My dreams are amazing while I'm bleeding; my subconscious speaks to me," she says. As an eating disorder survivor, her period is a reminder of her health and what she's overcome. "When it is close, I put my hands on my stomach and say, 'I love you, body. I am taking good care of myself. I love you for that.'"

Nicole, who dealt with bad menstrual cramps and migraines for over a decade, also resolved her issues through holistic methods. "I had menstrual pain that was based on a lack of care for the cycle," she explains. She took up self-care practices like abdominal massage, switched from tampons to menstrual cups and cloth pads, used hormone-balancing herbs and supplements, and eventually moved from New York City to a calm village in Portugal with access to nature. While herbs and massages may sound woo-woo, there's some data behind natural remedies like these, and doctors are even starting to recommend them.[8] Most importantly, they worked for Nicole, who hasn't gotten cramps in nine years. "I now experience painless menstruation and no longer have menstrual migraines," she says. Not only that, but her period enables self-discovery and body awareness. She enjoys tracking her cycle to prevent pregnancy and understand the changes she's experiencing. "I feel very clear-headed and ready to go into the next cycle," she says. "I also feel relief and enjoyment from menstruation. I'm actually able to feel the sensation of menstruation – what it feels like when blood exits without there being any actual cramping to it. My uterus will tell me when I'm about to menstruate. It sort of gently taps on my brain."

In a culture that pits women against their bodies, reclaiming menstruation helps Nicole exist in harmony with hers. "It's just the experience of living in my body that I enjoy," she says. "In this menstrual concealment society where we mostly like to cover up menses, I think it is very radical to actually embrace it and start to understand what it is that's going on. When I graduate from menstruation, I hope to have a lot of longevity and feel good in my body in menopause and perimenopause and pass down these traditions to younger menstruators – my nieces, even if I don't have a child myself. I think my role is to go through this whole completion of the menstrual life cycle and recognize it."

Bloody Hot Sex

Perhaps one reason period pleasures are taboo is that one such pleasure is – gasp – period sex. Many women, like me, enjoy it. A lot. The extra pelvic blood flow facilitates arousal and orgasm, and the blood provides natural lubrication.[9] "I know I'm not fertile at that time, so I can enjoy unprotected sex, and my partner and I can have closeness and intimacy," Nicole says. It's possible to get pregnant on your period, but by tracking her basal body temperature, cervical position, and cervical fluid, Nicole learned she has a "basic infertile pattern" that makes pregnancy unlikely during menstruation.[10] Meg loves period sex for different reasons:

> I didn't think I could have sex when I was on my period; I thought it was unhealthy, or there might have been some religious indoctrination in there. I realized, oh, I can, and it feels great! When my period starts, I am very, very horny, and different body parts feel like they have more nerve endings. So I tell my husband, "This week, focus on this body part." My breasts are extra sensitive in the best way possible. I want them to be kissed and touched and sucked and all the things. That is really only when I'm on my period. And it doesn't take as much time to reach orgasm. I want the orgasm faster, and I want him more.

These pleasurable experiences have helped Meg release ideas from her church about female pain as retribution for original sin. "There's no cursing in my opinion," she says. She now believes in a higher power that wants her to enjoy her period, sex, and her body. One that would tell her with pride: "Finally, you discovered this superpower that you have, and you're so fucking magical. And you didn't know it until you were thirty-three years old. And now you're rewriting the narrative, changing the dialogue, and telling other women: This isn't something to be feared."

Period Neutrality

The period positivity movement aims to destigmatize and celebrate menstruation. But not everyone feels period-positive. For those with health issues causing menstrual pain, positivity around menstruation may feel forced. And some period-positive advocates paint menstruators as feminine goddesses – another alienating idea for many women along with trans and non-binary people. Some menstrual supply brands and influencers claim periods connect us with the moon or signal women's motherly, cyclical nature. For those who resonate with these notions, they can be empowering. Any positive menstrual experiences are worth celebrating. But these ones are not universal.

What would menstruation look like if we saw it neither as a curse nor through the lens of forced positivity or stereotypes? For some, it could look how it does for me. I don't loathe my period, nor do I embrace it as an expression of feminine energy. Nor do I see it as something I *must love or else I'm not a feminist*. There are positives (orgasms) and negatives (leaks). It's only come with cramping when I've had other health issues, probably due to inflammation. Sometimes, I treat myself to chocolate or salt baths, as it's a nice invitation to up my dose of iron, magnesium, and pampering. But in general, I don't think much about it. I put on my period underwear and continue with my day. I'm more period-neutral than period-positive. In a world where our cycles weren't subject to pain or projections, more people could be.

Since we don't live in that world yet, we also must make space for those whose periods are unpleasant experiences. For them, the most pleasurable option may be to suppress menstruation. The fact that period pain isn't normal or natural doesn't mean there's always a simple fix for it. There hasn't been one for Celia, so she got an IUD to lessen her bleeding. When that didn't stop her endometriosis pain, she opted for surgery to remove her uterus and fallopian tubes. When she shares this on Twitter, some people – professed feminists included – tell her she's bypassing the sacred pain of womanhood. As with childbirth, this is not a battle between alternative and mainstream medicine. It's a battle between accepting pain and envisioning better lives for women. Unfortunately, both Western medicine and natural living advocates are guilty of normalizing pain, Celia points out:

> Women are told repeatedly that we have high pain tolerances when the reality is, our pain is ignored and dismissed. And we don't get the care and treatment we need to just be in less pain. We see this a lot with the "natural" movement – the way a lot of people (and women in particular) treat hormonal birth control or pain meds for childbirth. It's like it's a bad thing to not want to be in pain and it's natural or good to feel it. It's all bullshit. There's a lot of internalized misogyny in telling women they have to feel their pain and just be "natural." And of course, it all goes back to having children, right? Many of the treatments for pelvic pain involve not having a menstrual cycle, which means not having children or at least pausing that ability. At the end of the day, women still can't shake that expectation that we're supposed to be mothers and have children and we shouldn't interfere with that process, regardless of if we want children or not.

Nobody should face judgment in the name of period positivity. We should support women alleviating pain and enabling pleasure however they can. Yes, we must challenge the notion that all periods are painful and pleasureless. But we must also help all women create better bodily experiences for themselves. It doesn't matter if the means through which they do so are alternative or conventional. What matters is that we offer others, not fire and brimstones, but a hand to put the fire out. Nobody's house deserves to burn down.

Period-less Pleasure

Older women are subject to their own curse: the valuing of young, reproductively eligible women above them. And so menopause, like menstruation, has been defined by unpleasant symptoms. But in Joan's experience, it's much more. "I loved menopause," she says. "I could start wearing my white pants again. I didn't have to worry about being prepared for being bloody. I didn't have PMS anymore." Though hot flashes and night sweats – known as vasomotor symptoms – are seen as synonymous with menopause, a minority of 16–40% of women globally report moderate to severe vasomotor symptoms. Ninety percent report being untroubled by menopause, and 42% feel relief.[11] Like so many female experiences, menopause is made worse by disparaging views of it. Women with negative attitudes toward aging face more intense symptoms, while those from Asian cultures that emphasize respect for elders report fewer symptoms.[12] Racism and classism also impact menopause, with Black women experiencing worse and longer-lasting vasomotor symptoms than White women in the US, especially if they also have more stress and less education.[13]

As with periods, positive experiences with menopause get obscured behind the negative. Upsides include enjoying sex without pregnancy concerns and eliminating menstrual health issues. Uterine fibroids tend to shrink, resolving symptoms like urinary urgency and backaches.[14] But it goes deeper: Joan has come to live more for herself. During their reproductive years, women are expected to devote their lives to children or partners. But after menopause, a shift happens, Joan explains:

We start wanting to take care of ourselves more, and I think that's very good for us. We as women have often been taking care of other people most of our lives, and to reach the point where we can say "it's time for me now" is very important. In my gym, there are many other women in the locker room who would talk about that and say, "I told him to make his own damn dentist appointment." And everybody would laugh because we all knew just what she was talking about.

Once we stop apologizing for our bodies and our womanhood, we can adopt this attitude at any age. We can embrace the life stage we're in by giving fewer hoots how society defines us. Joan's advice? "Be authentic. Find what matters to you, and do what matters to you. Let go of the things that don't matter anymore. Let go of what other people think, what other people expect of you. Know that you are of value and you still have more to give. More to learn."

Chapter 12

No Pleasure, No Gain

Amanda struggled through painful sex for months without a solution in sight. She finally confided in her roommate, who said sex hurt her too. Over time, she developed a conspiracy theory: What if women's bodies weren't designed to enjoy intercourse, and men had duped them into thinking they did for their own benefit? She grew furious as she entertained the prospect that she'd been lied to about women's bodies her whole life. It turned out she *had* been told lies about women. But their enjoyment of sex wasn't one of them.

"I never thought of myself as being particularly undereducated about sexual things," she reflects. "I never thought of myself as a prudish person, so I thought I knew the necessary information already, but I did not." At first, she figured it was normal to be "sore" and her body was "just getting used to it." This was how the hymen worked, right? Never mind that this had gone on far too long for that to be the issue. She didn't tell her doctor out of fear of judgment. "I thought of gynecologists as people who were supposed to tell you to not have sex because that's pretty much what authority figures had told me growing up," she says. Eventually, after talking to other women and doing online research, it hit her: She had pain because she lacked pleasure. She hadn't known she should be turned on before intercourse. How would she? Porn depicted foreplay as kissing and perhaps a blowjob. Though few people expect men to attempt penetration without erections, that's basically what's expected of women. "I don't think I knew about the fact that vaginas change in size and stuff and need encouragement to do so," says Amanda. "I just don't think I realized that was a necessary part of intercourse because at least at that time, it was never shown in TV or movies. It was always, they make out and then they're having sex. And I guess that was where I got most of my sex ed. I remember feeling like something was wrong with me."

Without Pleasure, What's Left Is Pain

It's because we don't value women's pleasure that so many endure pain. The clitoris is seen as a bonus little button with no important role. Scientists characterize it as an evolutionary accident akin to male nipples, existing because the penis does.[1] Yet without it, women would have trouble feeling motivated or excited for sex. The clitoris may be "just for fun," but without fun, there's little room for enthusiastic consent. That makes the clit the most vital organ there is. Without pleasure, what's left is pressure. What's left is coercion. What's left is pain. By stigmatizing pleasure, we set women up for painful lives.

Amanda had to be proactive to receive enough pleasure to prevent pain. She aimed to orgasm before penetration to relax her pelvic muscles and ensure she was aroused. "After discovering that most women can't actually have an orgasm from just intercourse alone, I felt like I had been lied to my whole life," she says. "These women in the movies, they enjoy it so much. They're having orgasms. They don't show the part where they are having their clitoris stimulated." Part of it was also psychological; the discomfort got into a cycle. She'd get so anxious about pain due to her previous attempts, she'd tense up, and that would create more pain. Some women may experience this cycle simply from hearing horror stories about the hymen. Or from feeling pushed or rushed into sex. "I think the first time I had sex, I was really nervous," says Amanda. "It was kind of a procedural thing; it wasn't like we wanted to do it right then. We had planned to do it, so it didn't really happen in an organic way. I wasn't super in the mood, so that detracted from the experience a lot." Half the battle was "making sure I was actually in the mood and not feeling pressured," she says. Once she caught on to the difference that enthusiasm makes, she stopped having sex she didn't desire fully.

The other piece was gaining basic sexual health information. Amanda's sex ed was not abstinence-only but "abstinence is best," she says, imparting the message that "all sex is bad" and "you're kind of asking for it if something bad happens." It's no wonder it didn't ring alarm bells when sex *was* bad for her. Since all she'd learned was that sex could have negative consequences like pregnancy and STIs, she had to learn for herself how to make it positive. "At some point, we discovered lube, and that was a game changer," she recalls. Imagine if Amanda's school had taught her sex should feel pleasurable and safe. Imagine if her mom had taught her about the clitoris, consent, and lube instead of saying God would disapprove of her. Imagine if, instead of fearing adolescents will have sex and depriving them of information, we instead appropriately feared they'd have *painful* sex – and taught them how to prevent it.

Creating Positive Experiences Through Positive Words

So that women like Amanda need not figure things out on their own, educators are spreading the word that painful sex is preventable. Some are even changing the language we use to describe our anatomy. Sexual health sites like *Scarleteen* and *Our Bodies, Ourselves* use the term "vaginal corona" as an alternative to "hymen," reminding us there's no barrier to be broken.[2] Hopefully, as young people stop learning they have a "cherry" to "pop," they'll stop accepting sex that hurts. "Virginity" is another word experts are reexamining. One definition of virginity loss, introduced in Jessica Valenti's *The Purity Myth*, is having your first orgasm with a partner.[3] This is more empowering than defining virginity by the hymen but can discount sex that's not goal-oriented. Others have suggested we replace "virginity" with "sexual debut," a term popularized by sex educator Nicolle Hodges.[4] One playful tweet reads: "Losing/taking virginity turns sex into an object, places pressure on the decision, [and] you don't actually lose or take anything," while "sexual debut" is "exciting, all focus is on you, [and] suggests a musical number is involved."[5] Orchestra or dance notwithstanding, any word that denotes celebration instead of loss can help us see first-time sex as a gain. Not a pain through which future gain can come.

I don't mind the term "virginity," but it need not apply exclusively to penis-in-vagina sex. First-time intercourse is worth celebrating if we want, but so are lots of sexual and romantic experiences. I like to think of "virginities," plural. There's your kissing virginity, your dating virginity, your relationship virginity, your vibrator virginity, your shower sex virginity, your same-sex-encounter virginity, your sexting virginity. Compiling a list of virginities you look forward to losing – or rather winning – and checking off items as you find the right people is much more fun than demarcating one act as a transition from innocence to corruption. Everyone can define or not define virginities for themselves, including LGBTQ people who may always remain "virgins" in heteronormativity's eyes. Having a penis in your vagina need not mean you are changed. But you can get excited about all the changes that happen over your sexual lifespan. The most exciting part is, you'll never run out of milestones to mark. And with each one, you remain innocent. Nothing gets taken from you.

Preventing Pain Pleasurably

I never had pain with sex – not the first time, not ever. Since many have, I've thought about what made my experience different. I don't think I did anything special. More than anything, I stayed true to myself. I didn't cave to pressure to have sex before I was ready. I waited until I was halfway through college, with someone I trusted and desired. I'd used internal toys, so penetration was not new or scary. I did not experience pain or bleeding when I first used an insertable vibrator, but the fact that I was by myself helped me feel secure and go at my own pace. It also helped me see penetration as something that could be for my pleasure. And when I chose to share that with someone else, I wanted it – a lot. I honored my boundaries and timeline – something that should be a given but unfortunately isn't in our culture. I'd recommend that women – and everyone – wait to have sex until the prospect excites them. Physically and emotionally. No matter how excited your partner is, wait until you are. Making concessions will deprive you both of the greatest gift you can give: your sexual truth. Your genuine enthusiasm and pleasure. Everyone benefits when those things are present.

I also consulted another source – the sex advice column *Go Ask Alice* – which confirms my thinking that more pleasure is the path toward less pain. The column suggests fingering yourself (fun) well before you plan to have intercourse, gradually working up to more fingers. This way, if the corona partially covers your vaginal opening, it will stretch out comfortably. Make sure this is enjoyable for you; play with your clitoris too if that feels better. The column reads:

> Place a finger into your vagina (you can slick it up first with lube) and apply pressure on the vaginal entrance by pressing downward toward the anus. Keep the pressure on for a few minutes, and then release it. Repeat this procedure several times, each time with a little more pressure. Then insert two fingers and apply pressure to the sides of the vaginal entrance, in addition to the downward stretching. You can repeat this process over several days.[6]

Women really don't have to jump through hoops to avoid painful sex. Nor need we temper our expectations. It's time to expect more from our sex lives, not less. All the things I'm describing – self-pleasure, exploration, consent, communication, mutuality – are basic and doable. They would be a given in a healthy sexual culture. But we don't live in one, so I'm taking the space to lay them out here. Hopefully one day, as women go into first-time sex, the questions on their minds will sound less like "how do I avoid pain?" and more like "where can they touch me to turn me on?" or "what positions sound most exciting?" or "how can we set the mood to make it even more incredible?" But if that's not where we are yet, I'm happy to give some advice on how to get there. Especially if that advice involves sex toys.

Pain Is Not the Entrance Fee to Pleasure

Up until my sexual debut at twenty, I expected sex to hurt. Despite my intuitions otherwise, other women convinced me I was wrong. They said expecting only pleasure was a recipe for disappointment. So on the night it spontaneously happened, as The National hummed from my sticker-covered MacBook,

I told my boyfriend, "Please stop if it hurts me." I was terrified it would. I braced myself. I held my breath. I waited for pain. And waited. Why did it just feel ... fantastic? Finally, when I realized it was happening, I exclaimed through laughter, "That feels really good!" I'd had a hunch my body was not built to suffer through such a connective, joyful act. Now I knew this deep knowing was right. My self-trust grew. But I also oddly felt a bit guilty. Like I'd missed out on the romance of sacrificing my body for a partner, having him take something from me. Had I bypassed a rite of passage women had to traverse to become sexual? No pain, no gain, right? I'd experienced gain without pain. Did I deserve delight when I hadn't paid my dues?

Somewhere in my subconscious, I'd believed pain was the entrance fee to pleasure. That sorrow was the passageway to ecstasy. And this belief extended beyond sex. It came out in other ways: being scared to eat delicious food even if it was also nutritious because I couldn't comprehend it could be both. Hesitating to do homework for classes I liked because it didn't feel like homework – so how productive could it be? Taking a job on Friday nights because going out felt indulgent. Staying up late studying until I'd earned my sleep. Working extra hard after days off to compensate for my laziness. These were ways of hoarding pain so I could one day cash it in for pleasure. I delayed that day, as there was no amount of strain that felt sufficient to trade in for all the joy I craved.

To reject "no pain, no gain" is a paradigm shift that alters one's approach to life. To declare that the passageway to pleasure can *be pleasure* challenges mind-body dualism, puritanism, and hypercapitalism. Society's approach to work, food, rest, and money is fraught with "no pain, no gain." If we taught "no pleasure, no gain," we could free so many from the shackles of their mistreated bodies. We could dismantle painful labor: painful reproduction and painful toil. We could see enthusiastic consent as a prerequisite for any task. We could see play as a component of the workday. We could realize pleasure is part of health, not its enemy. We could view self-care as a foundation, not an indulgence. That's what paradise looks like, and pain is not its entrance fee. Its doors are already open to all.

Chapter 13

In Joy Thou Shalt Bring Forth Children

Debra, who spent her painful first birth in a hospital monitored by pushy staff, later gave birth joyfully at a midwife center. "I had midwives and people I felt safe with – people who didn't second-guess what I wanted," she says. "It felt completely different." She had a tub and shower for relaxation, a birth ball and stool to sit or lean on for comfort, a queen-sized bed to lie down, and essential oil emitting a soothing lavender scent. "When you go into that environment, it's like a mini retreat," she says. "It's easier to find pleasure in the experience." By that point, she understood "how birth was experienced on a physical level, but there was also an emotional, spiritual, and sexual component," she explains.

> By being in a birth center and having more options to find comfort than most hospitals offer, that birth was orgasmic. And I wouldn't at any point call it painful. It was intense. It was amazing. Being fully aware of how to move my body, I gave birth upright. Feeling my baby move through my body, and that moment of release – consciously being able to feel those last kicks and wiggles and feel his head as he was

moving out of me – that was orgasmic but not sexual at all. That incredible connection and that deep love release, that was so exquisite.

Even those who see painful periods and sex as avoidable may be skeptical that women can overcome the most normalized form of female suffering: childbirth pain. So let me acknowledge the elephant in the room: Debra's birth was not like most people's. Still, hearing stories like hers helps us learn how they *can* become more people's experience. When I impart accounts of pleasurable births, I preface them by saying: These are not standards to judge yourself against. There are many wonderful resources to make your ideal birth more likely, but there are few guarantees. There's a lot outside our control, and today's world isn't set up for everyone to have an easy birth. What I have seen, however, is that you can find elements of pleasure and joy in almost any birth. And I'm sharing these stories because, as I said, it's important to not just lament the present but lay out a new vision for the future. After all, it is the future we are birthing.

Embodying Ecstasy

Debra calls what she experienced an orgasmic birth. Orgasmic birth doesn't just mean having an orgasm during childbirth, known sometimes as a "birth-gasm." That happens too, but orgasmic birth is broader. It's a movement to allow for pleasure in birth, both physical and emotional. "We define 'orgasmic birth' to honor the people who have birth-gasms, but it's also for the people who find joy and pleasure and empowerment in birth in their own way," Debra explains. "A pleasurable birth is everybody's birthright – and would be possible if we supported people to give birth in whole new ways with a lot of available options for everyone to find comfort." We don't yet know how common orgasmic births are. One survey of 109 French midwives found their clients reported sexual pleasure in one in 300 births.[1] The true number may be higher, since not everyone will tell their midwife they orgasmed. And many women in the study used epidurals, which blunt pelvic sensation. When midwife Ina May Gaskin surveyed 151 mothers she knew, most of whom birthed at a midwife center, one fifth described their births as orgasmic.[2] So, while orgasmic births may be rare, they could be more common in optimal environments.

Ecstatic birth is a related movement emphasizing childbirth's potential for bliss. Meghan Hindi, a mother in New Jersey, describes one of her births as ecstatic but not orgasmic: "It took me to the stars and back." Ayelet remembers her two births as ecstatic too: "I was hysterically laughing." There's a fine line between ecstatic and orgasmic births, as "orgasmic" is not always sexual. "It was like a semi-orgasm," Ayelet laughs. "There were definitely components of orgasm in my births. I mean, orgasm comes in different waves and shapes and colors. So I would say there was something like that feeling of ecstasy when you peak in an orgasm. That's what labor is for me. It was that peak of ecstasy. It's like a wave that washes over me. It wasn't targeted to one area; it was like a full-body orgasm." Setting was crucial for Ayelet, who gave birth at her home in Jerusalem. "Being in my bed – in my space with my candles and my oils – just felt so much more natural for me," she says. While many ecstatic births take place in midwife centers or homes for calm and control, they don't have to. Most techniques for facilitating pleasure – music, massage, breathwork, aromatherapy, partner touch and support, birth balls, varied positions – can be brought to hospitals. "I don't think everybody's meant to have a home birth," says Ayelet. "For some women, I know they feel much safer in a hospital – in which case I say, birth where you feel safe."

Blessing Births

Ngozi hoped to hire a midwife when she first gave birth. "As a sexual abuse survivor, it was very important to me to have as much control in labor as possible," she says. But her friends told her midwifery was a "White hippie" practice that wouldn't accommodate Black women. She grew comfortable going to a midwife center when she learned of the US's long tradition of Black midwives. "Without knowing our history, we may not understand that midwifery is not new to us," she explains. During her five births, Ngozi not only experienced "euphoria" but began viewing her body as powerful instead of helpless due to her past abuse. "I realized my body, which I believed was broken, could do amazing things," she says. "Breastfeeding was a continuation of that – that sense of empowerment that my breasts, which at one time were ugly and distorted, were able to feed my children. As a child, I was told that birth was the most horrible thing ever and there wasn't anything positive about birth. So I'm glad I was able to overcome that and change the narrative and tell clients: Birth can be really frickin' awesome no matter your background."

In recent years, a resurgence of doulas and midwives has offered parents a positive lens to view childbirth through.[3] Midwives – health professionals trained in obstetric care – use fewer medical interventions than doctors and work in centers and homes as well as hospitals. Doulas are more like birth companions, offering education, advocacy, emotional support, and assistance with natural comfort techniques. Women who employ doulas have 39% fewer C-sections, 15% more uninduced vaginal births, and 35% fewer negative experiences.[4] Some parents can move beyond the curse of childbirth thanks to providers who believe in their blessedness – their capability and strength. "I distinctly remember hearing one of my midwives tell me how beautifully I was bringing my baby down," writes mother Shalome Stone on the *Orgasmic Birth* website. "It was exactly what I needed to hear. I felt strong."[5] Even in her hospital birth, Debra's pain let up when her doctor told her, "You're doing it. You can do it." When we stop psyching parents out and give them tools to master birth, we halt the self-perpetuating cycle of fear and discomfort. In a 2021 study, just one class on relaxation methods brought mothers' pain levels down, sometimes to the point of not requesting medication.[6]

Once we liberate women from the myth of sorrowful birth, their joy and comfort grow. Those with less fear report more positive births and fewer C-sections and instrumental deliveries.[7] "If you're able to trigger the relaxation reflex rather than the fight-or-flight response, then you get a positive feedback loop between oxytocin and endorphins," explains midwife Barbara Montani. One way to encourage this feedback loop is to incorporate pleasure into birth, whether it's sexual (e.g. touching your clitoris) or just sensual (receiving massage). Both these activities stimulate oxytocin and reduce pain perception.[8] As with painful sex, the stigma against pleasure contributes to painful childbirth. When we feel pleasure, less room is left for pain. Debra invites people seeking orgasmic births to consider the conditions under which they'd orgasm. "The same hormones of conception and orgasm are the same hormones that need to flow in labor," she says. "And if you look at the conditions in our current hospital environments, how many people would have great orgasms in them? Most people can't imagine an orgasmic birth because they have so much pain. If you have not tasted or experienced it, you can't imagine it. And the problem is, we're not educating people on all their options."

Opening to Intensity

The most common word parents use when I ask about their pleasurable births is "intense." They describe labor as intense but not painful. "My third birth was more like an intense workout, an intense challenge," says Debra. Ayelet explains her experience: "Is birthing painful? It's intense but not impossible. And I can very confidently say that the more aligned I was and aware of the mind-body connection and the more I kept telling my body what to do, the less intense the experience became and the more possible it became." Meghan puts it this way: "Think of intensity in food, spice, sensuality in the mouth. Intense Italian food is like the greatest orgasm in your mouth. You could even have intense chocolate – so much bliss. Then I could say, 'intense sex.' That can be a lot of things. It's usually pretty good, but it requires surrender and safety." For many, birth is similar, which is why some incorporate the same elements into birth that improve sex. Some hold, kiss, and caress their partners. Madison Young, author of *The Ultimate Guide to Sex Through Pregnancy and Motherhood*, self-pleasured with a Hitachi Magic Wand. "I wouldn't classify any part of my forty-seven-hour labor as painful," she says. "I experienced pleasure, ecstasy, complete surrender, and high levels of intensity during my labor, but never pain."

Since society ingrains in us that giving birth hurts, Ayelet made a conscious choice not to expect pain. "If I label labor as painful, then my brain is going to process it as painful," she says. "It's going to actually send signals to my nerves saying 'this is a painful experience' – in which case, when a person's in pain, what do we do? We constrict our bodies, and there's a channel the baby has to go through. If that channel is constricted because the woman is in pain, it makes it that much more challenging for the baby to come out with ease, grace, and flow."[9] The first step to unwinding the curse, then, is acknowledging the possibility that intense sensations can be a blessing. For some, it is intensity that enables ecstasy.

Birthing Joyful Lives

Birth workers sometimes say we birth the way we live. The more presence, joy, and embodiment we live with, the more available pleasure is to us while birthing. Meghan made a point to slow down and get into nature to prepare for birth, and she maintains these habits for an ecstatic life. "It starts with a lifestyle that is more geared toward pleasure," she reflects. "I make fresh bread and teach my kids how to cook fresh food. Even if you're in an urban environment, you can learn to experience pleasure and deep mindfulness – not in a hippie sense but a human sense."

For Amber Hartnell, whose orgasmic, painless twelve-hour labor appeared in Debra's *Orgasmic Birth* documentary, the key was welcoming strong sensations fearlessly. To birth and live without strain, Amber has practiced saying "yes" to the moment and staying present with intense experiences rather than seeking escape. This can mean sitting and breathing deeply with challenging emotions instead of distracting yourself, or even learning to enjoy physically intense experiences like ice baths (just not while pregnant).[10] "Everything we experience is all sensation," says Amber. "It's how we choose to translate that sensation. We keep replicating what we've been taught, what we've been modeled. We can train ourselves to develop new neural pathways where we can stay completely in our bodies and not leave ourselves. Most people, when they're in the flood of intense sensations, the tendency is to contract away from it, to feel overwhelmed, to think 'I can't handle this.' On the other side of the resistance is a profound release, and in that release can be an experience of profound ecstasy." But acceptance does not mean passivity. Ayelet applied what she'd learned studying meditation to gain control over her thoughts:

I learned how to focus my mind on whatever the task is at hand. That awareness alone made it blissful and caused me to absolutely crack up during labor. My mom thought I was high. It's so easy to focus on the pain or the intensity or the sensations in the body that are uncomfortable, and then the mind starts to anticipate the next contractions and we don't give our bodies time to rest in between the waves. But there is time in between each contraction. If we take advantage of that time, then we're actually giving the body that strength to ride the next wave once it comes. I also kept telling myself: Every wave, every contraction doesn't last more than one minute. I can do anything for one minute, no matter how intense. I just kept telling myself: By the end of this, I'm going to hold my baby.

Ayelet describes birth as a conversation between her mind and body, a dance between surrender and control. "You can't totally shut off the mind and surrender to the body," she says. "The control center, which is in the brain, tells the body how to navigate. For example, if I'm in yoga and I'm in pigeon pose and I say 'ooh, I'm tight in my right hip,' I can start by feeling into the body, just feeling the sensations that are there. But then it requires the mind to be like 'OK, you can relax a little more. You're OK. You can surrender.' And the moment I tell myself in my brain 'you can surrender,' my right hip opens a little more, relaxes a little more." The same thing happened during birth: She let her body do what it needed while reminding it she was safe.

Discovering a Brand New Body

Discussions of postpartum life tend to focus on recovering from the pain of birth. But childbirth can open someone up to a more ecstatic state of being. "My ability to experience pleasure amplified," says Amber. "Birth is really an opportunity for a woman to be initiated into a whole other level of power and drop so deeply into her center and her intelligence." Giving birth "helped me see the power of myself, of my body, my womanness," Meghan echoes. As a sexual abuse survivor, this was healing:

> I felt so strong, so in control of my body. Not in control, *one with*. My body was in control, and when it wanted to go wild, I went wild with it. It gave me so, so much peace and strength. I remember pushing her out. I was moaning and breathing, and I looked up at my midwives as my legs were open and my breasts were out, and I winked at them. I was like, "We're doing this thing, yeah!" We were all giggling and laughing and the music was pounding, and then I reached down as her head came out and touched her head. And I said, "Hi, baby, hi!" I was claiming the moment for myself when I couldn't before. I was amazed by how blissful and not painful it was. And I stayed there. I was present the whole time because I didn't dissociate. I didn't remove myself from my body. I didn't need to. And that was the birth that just shook everything: I was no longer what they said I was. I was no longer what they did to me. In that moment, I was like Asherah, the empowered and primal life-giving queen of heaven.[11] I labored under my trees with my animals, roared at the mountain in my tub, and giggled as I opened wide to give fearless birth under the sun and sky. It's so joyful. It's so pure, that birth energy. It's like the greatest peace and safety your inner child can find.

This birth removed emotional blockages impacting every area of Meghan's life. Creative inspiration flooded her afterward. Without thinking, she sat down and wrote her first book with her child still at her breast. "I did not believe I was capable of writing a book or becoming an entrepreneur or doing the incredible things that I did and am still doing," she says. Able to hear her intuition more acutely, she began trusting her instincts to protect her daughters and raise her son to be a good man – two things she was scared she couldn't do because of her trauma.

Not everyone's postpartum experience is this exuberant. But while postpartum depression is common, it stems from lack of support, difficult births, low self-esteem, poverty, trauma, and other external sources more than hormones. "Hormonal changes occur in all those experiencing pregnancy and childbirth, and yet only some people experience emotional distress or poor mental health at these times," says women's health researcher Sally King.[12] Once again, it's not women's bodies but the world around them that's causing their problems. If we valued connection and community and helped people care for their families, more could enjoy parenthood as a blessing. Not just for their kids, but for themselves. "I felt more connected to my body," says Ngozi. "I was more in tune with where my vaginal muscles were." This led her sex life to improve after childbirth. Postpartum sex, in fact, can feel like discovering a brand new body. After the first few months of recovery, when parents can explore non-penetrative acts, some unearth novel capabilities like squirting or orgasming through intercourse. The repositioning of pelvic nerves invites them to discover their sensual selves for the very first time all over again.[13]

Reverent Pleasure in the Uprightness of Women

No, women are not cursed with sorrowful childbirth. Yes, we have the potential for it. But we also possess the potential to bring forth children in joy. To parent in joy. To live in joy. Why, then, has women's vast potential for empowering, pleasurable births been squandered? Perhaps because people don't trust women to lead the process. From doubting of sexual assault victims to medical gaslighting to reproductive rights restrictions, women are constantly distrusted. Is it any wonder that when it comes to childbirth, we're deprived of decision-making?

When I presented this theory to Ayelet, she had a slightly different take. "I don't know if it's that they inherently don't trust women," she said. "It's that men trust women too much that it scares them because it puts women in the driver's seat. We saw it in the 1500s when they were burning witches and healers at the stake. Women were the medicine women. They were the healers, they were the magicians, they were the sorcerers – and men were like, 'What is going on? It's a threat to our sovereignty.'" Though the myth of women's cursedness is prevalent, it's so clearly false, people still don't believe it. If we really believed women were cursed, we wouldn't work so hard to tamp down their blessings. The view of women as designed for pain serves to undermine the power of their pleasure. But that power can't be denied, as Meghan so eloquently puts it:

> It's right there, but we shut it down. It's the power of "yes" over and over again until you feel yourself splitting – not literally, but that's how it feels: Your hips open. Out comes a new life. The power of "yes" pushes that head out, and that final "yes" is literally capable of creating a new human being that goes on to impact our world forever. But meanwhile, the world is too busy telling women to not be so loud, to not make their own choices, to be of profit to the system, to not question the intentions of those in power. What if instead of getting off on a woman on her knees being of service as a sexual object, what if as a society, we started seeking reverent pleasure in the uprightness of women breaking into a hundred pieces only to be reborn, expand, and create new life?

Chapter 14

I Will Greatly Multiply Thy Orgasms

Sammi was just about ready to give up. At forty-six, she'd never had an orgasm. She thought her clitoris looked small, so maybe she was biologically destined for pleasurelessness. Then, in a last-ditch effort to revitalize her sex life, she made her way to one of sex educator Betty Dodson's Bodysex workshops, where women gathered to talk about sex and masturbate. She felt broken during "genital show and tell" as she saw what looked like better-designed, better-functioning vulvas on the other participants. But Dodson's assistant Carlin Ross had a feeling Sammi's problem stemmed from somewhere else. Her husband shamed her interest in kink, and she'd never had a chance to explore it. So, as the women masturbated, Carlin conducted a little experiment and described domination and submission fantasies to Sammi. Before long, she'd had her first orgasm. Then her second. "See, you're normal," Carlin told her. "You're just not vanilla."

Sammi realized then and there that her body was not the problem. *She* was not the problem. When she shared her awakening with her husband, he felt threatened by her kinkiness, bisexuality, and empowerment. She finally saw she was more than capable of sexual satisfaction – just not with him. They separated soon after, and after meeting a kink-positive man, she orgasmed the first time he touched her supposedly inadequate clitoris. During their fourth rendezvous, she orgasmed ten times from his hands, a vibrator, and intercourse. "Seems I just needed what I needed," she concludes.

It's Normal to Get Off Every Time

Women aren't stopping at eliminating pain. They have a hunch about their capacity for pleasure, and they won't stop until they enjoy it. Nor are Dodson and Ross the only advocates unveiling women's orgasmic potential. Artist Sophia Wallace creates posters with "laws of cliteracy" ("clitoral literacy") like "a man would never be expected to get off through sex acts that ignored his primary sexual organ," "freedom in society can be measured by the distribution of orgasms," and – my favorite – "masturbating inside women is not sex."[1] When she speaks at colleges, young women sometimes worry female orgasms are too much trouble. "Nope," she tells them. "It's normal to get off *every* time. Like, four or five times." Some may see this as setting up unrealistic expectations. But as I said, it's time women expect more, not less, from sex and life. As another cliteracy print reads, "Raise your standard of sexual entitlement to include multiple orgasms and no pain."[2] Such standards only seem unrealistic due to male-centered conditioning and habituation to the status quo. Women should "never settle for a sexual relationship where they aren't having regular pleasure with orgasms," Wallace says.

> Part of why I think this is happening so regularly is that women and femmes have been socialized to define their happiness around the satisfaction of someone else. We have been taught to deprioritize our own sexual satisfaction to the extent that many women are in relationships with men they are not

sexually attracted to. This is tragic if you think about it. We have been socialized to know how to be objects of desire, but we're still alienated from our own embodied pleasure and the speaking up required to experience it. Additionally, quite a few heterosexual men are not working hard to stay sexy for their partners. While women are under constant pressure to be hot from girlhood, men do not live with an existential sense of precarity if they do not maintain attractiveness to straight women. I wish I could change the mindset of so many women from "if I'm lucky I'll get off too" to "I only have sex with people I am attracted to and who sexually please me." And one more thing: Slut shaming is so outdated. If anyone should be shamed, it is narcissexuals, those hoarders of orgasms who take and then leave everyone unsatisfied.

As a queer woman, Wallace says the "elusive female orgasm" narrative just doesn't exist in her community. Nor does the idea that women should "just enjoy the journey" and "let go" of the destination. "The vast, vast majority of people with this anatomy from a very young age with the correct stimulation – let's just say a decent vibrator – will consistently orgasm pretty quickly all the time," she argues. "The idea of taking an orgasm out of the equation is totally absurd, and it's really lazy. It's inexcusable to make that somehow extra." For a woman to have lots of orgasms is normal and expected in her circle. It should be everywhere. Even among women like Sammi who are preorgasmic – i.e. have never orgasmed – the vast majority can learn. In one study, 90% of preorgasmic women had their first orgasms within three months of receiving sex therapy and doing at-home self-pleasure exercises, with 85% orgasming in three-quarters or more of their partnered encounters.[3] University of Florida professor and sex therapist Laurie Mintz, author of *Becoming Cliterate*, tells me every preorgasmic woman she's worked with has learned to orgasm, except one hindered by antidepressants.[4]

Like Wallace, Mintz likes to challenge young women's perceptions of their limitations. At the start of each semester, she surveys students on their sex lives. In the beginning, the women expect sex to be orgasmless and sometimes painful. But after she helps them understand the importance of clitoral stimulation and arousal before penetration, women start having more orgasms and less pain. "It has this ripple effect in their life," she says. "They just feel better about themselves in general. If you're unhappy in your sex life, you have this shame, and you feel crappy about yourself. It just kind of gives you that overall bounce in your step." We could all use that bounce. We could all stand to let go of that shame. We could all stand to define our bodies by what they can do, not what they can't.

"Very Powerful But Barely Acknowledged"

Hida, who is intersex, used to "hit a wall" during sex. "I had to stop right before it felt like I was going to orgasm because it felt like I would urinate," s/he recalls. At a friend's suggestion, s/he tried masturbating while focusing on physical sensations and tuning out mental chatter. "I was thrilled that it worked," Hida remembers. "I actually didn't 'have issues having an orgasm,' as I'd started to believe, and I quickly started having multiple orgasms of all kinds during sex as well. Not only that, but years later, I shared this information during a female sexuality course – and several fellow students later told me that they tried it and it had worked for them too: They'd had their first orgasms. What this tells me is that many women are probably not experiencing orgasms for the same reason: They are letting their minds get in the way – and I think this is perfectly natural in a culture that discourages and even shames female sexuality. So these beliefs are ingested by women and limit females' ability to orgasm, which in turn reinforces the belief that the female orgasm is elusive."

A well of pleasure bursts open and overflows when we overcome self-consciousness and embrace how our bodies respond. "I later learned that this feeling of needing to urinate is actually very typical right before female ejaculation, another form of female orgasm that is very powerful but barely acknowledged," says Hida. "So what I had been experiencing when I felt like I needed to urinate was physically perfectly normal – I just hadn't known it, as most still don't. It all makes me think about how much more joyful and empowered all females could be if educated about their own sexuality." Hida's realization about "the immense sexual pleasure available to females via the clitoris" helped he/r see "how much the efforts to remove this empowered female sexuality are revealed and enforced by the practice of clitoral reduction surgeries," s/he explains. "These are performed right here in the US on children who have ovaries, are girls (and later women), menstruate, and can get pregnant but simply happen to have large clitorises. My empowered, multi-orgasmic, life-enhancing sexual experiences would not be possible without my abundant female sex organ – and it is very clear that societal attitudes attempt to prevent this very experience due to misogyny, sexism, and homophobia." It really is the fear of our blessings that leads others to treat us as cursed, whether by trying to change female and intersex bodies or simply deeming them flawed. Our biggest "flaws" are often our greatest gifts.

It's Raining Orgasms

The breakthrough that helped me have my first partnered orgasm came from sex therapist Vanessa Marin's online course "Finishing School." I didn't learn any elaborate new techniques – but I learned it was OK to ask partners for what I wanted. And to give myself what I wanted. Marin included a quote from the book *I Love Female Orgasm* in her lectures:

We can't tell you how many women have shared with us that the time their sex life blasted to a new level was when they started taking responsibility for their own orgasms. This is one area where women could stand to learn a thing or two from the guys. Guys don't lie back, waiting hopefully for their partners to give them an orgasm – they rub or thrust in just the way they like, at just the right speed for them, at just the right rhythm, at their favorite angle. Guys negotiate, ask, or set things up so they can have sex in their favorite positions, the ones that give them their favorite kind of physical or visual stimulation. Guys think the thoughts and fantasize the fantasies that turn them on while they're having intercourse. Guys make it clear that they expect to have lots of sexual pleasure, and an orgasm, and they assume the sexual interlude will continue until they do.[5]

As I listened, I asked myself: What had I been doing to advocate for my orgasms? Not much – because I thought they were elusive. I figured they were too much work. I assumed they'd take too long, although they didn't by myself. After all, they took twenty minutes with a partner, didn't they? Or was it forty-five? Whatever it was, it sounded daunting. But not so much anymore. I happened to be entering a new relationship, so I made up my mind to practice the "male" approach the next time my partner pleased me. Instead of giving up, I would do whatever worked. I already knew how. I just had to give myself permission to do what I did by myself. I followed through on that promise. I let him know it felt good when he touched my clitoris. I moved my body to keep his hand on the right spot. I spread my legs to provide more access. I let my mind enter all the freaky fantasies it conjured. I continued even as I grew afraid his hand would fall off. And as I thought maybe, just maybe I was close, I moaned and squeezed his arm to communicate *do not stop*. He didn't. Then it happened. Then again. Then, after a brief nap, again. When it rains, it pours, I thought – which is a pretty sweet deal when it's raining orgasms.

So much of my problem was self-fulfilling. The idea that female orgasms were elusive had discouraged me from trying to have one – and left me too anxious to focus when I did try. Once I stopped worrying about *not* climaxing, orgasming with my partner became easy and not time-consuming at all. I did every time we had sex for three years. And with each one, I got a piece of my soul back. I came to see my femaleness in a new way. I stopped defining myself by deficiency. And once I saw I was not inferior to men in sex, I saw I was not inferior to men in life. It was a lie. I saw that now: If my body wasn't really inferior, if I had been fooled about that, then I might have been fooled about my mind's inferiority too. I did not have to strive and strain to measure up to men. I did not have to fight to become equal. Nope. I was equal by design.

I continued working through my hangups with a sex coach, confessing my fear that I was complicated. "If you think you're complicated and you're worried about it, that might *make* sex complicated," he told me. Perhaps, I thought, that's what's happening to women writ large. We're taught we're complex, we're cursed, our pleasure is difficult to attain. And then we feel guilty for requesting the supposedly hard work of getting us off. So of course we neglect our needs. Of course we tense up in the bedroom. Of course it becomes harder to orgasm when you fear your pleasure is inaccessible. Anxiety is the number one obstacle to orgasm women report.[6] "But I don't think women are more complicated," my coach said. "I think women are more orgasmic. If reincarnation exists, I want to come back as a woman."[7] I no longer felt unfortunate to be one.

"I Was Never Broken"

Margaret's problem, too, did not stem from being female. After three years off her medication, her orgasms were not elusive anymore. "I just think my body needed that three years to flush out the SSRIs from my system and heal," she says. "I cried because it was so emotional. I felt like I had a missing piece of me back. Since then, I have gotten a lot more comfortable in my sex life and have found a very supportive partner." Still, her seven years unable to orgasm taught her something valuable. She learned to appreciate her body unconditionally, whether or not it performed the way she hoped. And through this appreciation, sex became less performative and more playful. "When this all started, I felt broken," she reflects. "But over time, I accepted my body and who I was. I learned to think of sex as less of a linear experience with a distinct end that made everything worth it, and more about connecting with another person. It's amazing that I can have orgasms and have mostly normal sexual function back, but I also recognize that I was a whole person that entire time. I was never broken or empty."

While Kaytlin now can orgasm through partnered sex, she's still learning how to do so consistently. She's also become gentler with herself about her struggles, mainly by realizing they're not hers alone. In her comedy show *Whore's Eye View*, she quips that for thousands of years, men were encouraged to "make their brides bleed on their wedding night – and then had the audacity to complain about how hard it is to make women come." I couldn't have said it better myself. It's understandable if we don't have pleasure at our fingertips when the world is set up for our pain. Yes, we are capable of orgasms and much more. And if we don't have that now, we haven't failed. We may not unravel the millennia-old curse on our bodies in days, weeks, or months. What we can do is take away the self-judgment that comes with it.

Why *do* so many women's orgasms seem elusive? Why do they seem to take a lot of time or warm-up? Why can they be unpredictable? Why are they sometimes absent if the mood's not right? Because an orgasm is the body's way of saying "yes." And right now, women have a lot to say "no" to. Not climaxing can be a way for the body to say "no." To a pushy lover. To a relationship that's not right. To an upbringing that shamed your sexuality. To a society that's marginalized your body. To a community where you cannot take up space. To a culture that undervalues your desire. To an environment your health cannot thrive in. Our pleasurelessness is not a condition set in stone, but like our pain, it is a message. It signals what's wrong with the world around us. And for that, it must be revered. It's a healthy response to an unhealthy world. This response lives in our bodies, but the shame and blame are not ours to carry. The curse is not ours to carry. And just knowing that is the first step toward shucking it off.

Chapter 15

Living Life Orgasmically

"I'm afraid the only option is to surgically remove part of your cervix."

Twenty-six-year-old Josefina stared blankly at the doctor in a daze as he explained her pre-cervical cancer diagnosis. The future she'd envisioned and worked toward, one that included motherhood and vibrant health, suddenly seemed bleak.

"Will that get rid of the problem?"

"It will for the time being, though the pre-cancerous cells could grow back."

"Well, what are the risks? Will I be able to have kids if I go through with it?"

"It's possible, but you'll have a 30% chance of miscarrying."

Josefina remembers feeling ashamed of her body at that moment. Like it had failed her. Like an organ she thought she could rely on to cultivate life and provide pleasure had instead spawned sickness and pain. Like the core of her womanhood was damaged.

"That doesn't sound like something I want to do," she said.

"Well, you don't have a choice," the doctor chuckled, making her feel even more embarrassed and small. Adrenaline coursed through her veins as she felt anger accumulated from years of men telling her what to do with her body. Her rage escalated as she learned her past four pap smears were abnormal, yet this doctor had done no further testing until now. But she wasn't ready to take his words as a given. Deep down, she had a hunch that removing part of her body wasn't the solution – because her body wasn't the problem. Her cervix was communicating a deeper problem. A problem with the way she'd treated herself, been treated by others, and been treated by society at large. She wanted to learn from her body, attend to it, honor it, and heal it on the deepest level, not shame the messages it was sending.

Creating a Whole New Choice

When Josefina was molested at eleven, she came to believe it was unsafe to be female. Her sexuality seemed dangerous and shameful. Because of that, she grew to view herself as unworthy of love. She had toxic relationships and unfulfilling sex to mask her feelings of worthlessness, which created more shame over being "promiscuous." She'd abandoned herself and disconnected from her body. And she knew if she did not address that, she would not fully heal. She was picking up on the increasingly substantiated truth that sexual trauma plays a role in physical illness, particularly pelvic illnesses. Yet Western medicine knows little about how to heal from the inside out. So, Josefina charted new territory as she did something she wished she'd done her whole life: listened to her body.

The first step she took to reconnect with her vessel was to make her own decisions around her health, not take her doctor's "no choice" assessment as gospel. He, like the man who molested her, had left her feeling powerless. She resolved to take her power back. She did her own research and consulted holistic doctors, then threw herself into healing methods that felt right to her, including eastern modalities and a naturopathic herbal treatment called escharotics.[1] "You think you can take my choice away?" she recalls thinking. "I created a whole new choice. I created a whole new road that you told me was not available." And while she was diligently planning her meals and taking supplements, Josefina worked to heal her sexuality. She studied yoga and meditation and developed a self-pleasure practice aimed at cultivating respect for her body. She discussed her sex life with mentors and came to understand how even some consensual experiences contributed to her self-abandonment, as she had not desired them 100%. As she explored tantra by herself and with caring partners, she began seeing the beauty in her sexuality rather than just the pain and trauma. She remembers realizing: "You're sacred, you're powerful, you can create magic. You have this life force within you, this sacred energy of the cosmos."

Emotional healing like this is no substitute for medical care. But sometimes, it's the missing link. Oncologist Kelly Turner, who studies unexpected cancer remissions, found that nearly all patients she followed who recovered from bleak cases had done what Josefina did. They listened to their intuitions, took control of their health, released suppressed feelings, deepened their spirituality, and did whatever helped them feel good.[2]

"A Complete Metamorphosis of Embodying Pleasure"

A year and a half after her diagnosis, Josefina returned to the doctor for a pap smear and found her pre-cancerous cells gone. Not only that, but where she was previously numb, she enjoyed newfound sensitivity and aliveness. "My pussy was like, 'Hello, girl, wake up,'" she smiles. As she continued studying sexuality and reconnecting with her body, she uncovered pleasure she never thought herself capable of. Not only could she feel the underwhelming orgasms she'd had earlier in life, but more parts of her body became orgasmic. "I went from experiencing pain and shame into a complete metamorphosis of embodying pleasure," she recounts. Even her cervix, previously a source of suffering, became her ally as she explored cervical orgasms.

Sophie's lightbulb moment arrived through a different route but led her down a similar path. After getting her masters in psychology thinking she'd become a therapist, she realized she wasn't in a place to guide others because she'd neglected her own well-being – particularly her sexual well-being. She had low self-esteem and poor boundaries, sought sex for validation, and didn't know how she wanted to be loved. Behind these struggles were negative sexual experiences and a lack of education about her body. She began working with a sex coach, who gave her self-pleasure practices to help her feel comfortable in her skin and reawaken dormant sensation. She also learned a practice called breathwork, which uses breathing exercises to tap into unfelt emotions.

"I remember my body would start kicking and saying 'no' and shaking to clear out any of these things that were stored there during breathwork, and with that, creating all this safety in myself: knowing I'm safe in my body, my body is mine, I can choose what's a 'yes' and a 'no,'" she recalls. As Sophie tuned in to her desires, she forewent sex that wasn't nourishing and uplifting. She'd assumed it would take lots of effort to orgasm with a partner; she'd have to battle against her body's dysfunction. But she simply had to shed layers of shame that were blocking her innate capacity. Her first partnered orgasm flowed naturally and unexpectedly, as her boyfriend was fingering her, when she decided *not* to try to climax. "What I realized was that it's not so much about learning certain techniques or tips to feel more pleasure, but it's about releasing the obstacles in the way," she says. "It was mostly about relaxation and acceptance of not really trying so hard. I had this whole story that there was something wrong with me. I felt not good enough because I wasn't able to do that. So it felt like a relief: Oh, see, I can do it! See, nothing's wrong with me."

The Tree of Knowledge of Good

Nothing was wrong with Sophie – and more was right than she imagined. As she continued working through her inhibitions, she learned to orgasm through intercourse, an ability she'd thought was reserved for a select few genetically blessed women. Many assume this, as clitoral orgasms are the usually lowest-hanging fruits. But there are many ways to stimulate the clitoris during intercourse – touching yourself, having a partner touch you, incorporating toys, using positions that enable grinding against a partner's body.[3] In one thirty-two-study meta-analysis in Elisabeth Lloyd's *The Case of the Female Orgasm*, 55% of women reported "usually, regularly, or always" orgasming through intercourse – a number that includes people who took advantage of these techniques.[4] Orgasms through penetration may also be enabled by the vagus nerve, which carries sensation from the vagina and cervix to the brain, and the inner clitoris, which wraps around the vagina. No type of orgasm is superior, and because of the inner clitoris, it's hard to separate "clitoral" and "vaginal" anyway. There aren't two clear-cut types of orgasms, but many areas that can elicit the brain's orgasmic response.[5] Once we stop hierarchizing them, we can non-judgmentally enjoy them all by themselves and when combined. Then, orgasms during intercourse become, not an obligation, but an invitation for exploration. Sophie considered them impossible, but as she processed trauma with patience and practiced penetration with toys, she surprised herself.

Through this exploration, Sophie discovered cervical orgasms, G-spot orgasms, and orgasms that felt like they had no center. "It's like a whole-body thing where I don't even really know where it comes from – it just starts to get a life of its own, and then it's hard to describe at that point," she says. Now a sex and relationship coach, she wonders how many women can feel pleasure in more ways than they believed but haven't had the chance to learn. After all, even in today's sexual culture, women delight in a variety of sensations. Half report experiencing both clitoral and vaginal orgasms, though many don't distinguish between "types" since multiple areas are often involved at once.[6] In one study, 86% of healthy women said vaginal stimulation contributed to their orgasms, and 46% said cervical stimulation played a role.[7] As many as 12% of women have orgasmed through breast stimulation, and 10% have experienced a "coregasm" – an orgasm achieved through exercise, as activating the abdominal and pelvic muscles can stimulate the surrounding nerves. Others can orgasm through stimulation of the neck or lips or even without physical touch, whether through vivid fantasizing, breathwork, or visual stimulation. These experiences induce the neurological and hormonal changes that typically accompany orgasm.[8] For me, touch-free orgasms are less pinpointed than genital ones but include a similar buildup and release of pleasure along with shaking or pulsating in the body.

Many women also experience multiple orgasms consecutively. For some, they're "rapid fire," each immediately following the other. But even those who don't have them so close together can often have more than one per session – and that counts too. Multiple orgasms are most common in healthcare professionals: 39% reported having them "usually or often" in one study, compared to 14% of the other women.[9] It's unlikely that women outside health professions are less biologically capable. Rather, the discrepancy is evidence that education makes a difference. Women who understand their bodies' capabilities have eaten from the tree of knowledge of good. Previously unsure whether multiple orgasms existed, Sophie now sometimes has trouble deciphering when one ends and the next begins. "It starts just kind of going into waves," she says. "Once I get there, I can just keep going on forever."

Life as One Giant Orgasm

Josefina likes to call herself "highly orgasmic" – and she is talking about more than sex. Her life feels like "one giant orgasm," a series of sensual delights. Pleasurable waves rush through her body when her partner touches her collarbone, the sensation of her shirt against her nipples teases her, and just drinking a cup of coffee is ecstatic. "I'm not depriving myself or feeling guilty for having pleasure but instead thinking, how good can I feel?" she says. The answer continues to surprise her. Eve has been falling for thousands of years, but she's returning to paradise. "To connect more with my body and tap into my own sexuality, it's almost like it unlocks a deeper ability to feel more alive and connected to everything," says Sophie. "I feel like I just literally opened up my body to sense more, to feel more, instead of being in protection mode. And when I'm able to tap into that, even days after, it stays in my body for a while. Colors are brighter, and I experience life in a much more alive way."

The orgasmic life is not just about physical pleasure; it's about reclaiming your right to well-being. Research finds time and time again that great sex makes women happier.[10] It makes sense: Orgasms release oxytocin, dopamine, and serotonin, promoting contentedness, connection, and calm.[11] But many describe something deeper: An about-face in how they view themselves. Discovering your pleasure potential can feel like no less than a discovery of your true self. The self that was there before sex-negativity and rape culture shrouded it. The self that was there before the fall. The self that has remained there, waiting to be uncovered, outlasting the shame that caused Eve to shroud her desire. We can rewrite this mythology in the privacy of our bedrooms, in the primacy of our bodies.

For Sophie, feeling the joy she'd long been denied challenged feelings of inadequacy that afflicted her for years. Knowing she was designed for an orgasmic life makes her "excited to be a woman," she says. And once she came to understand and appreciate what her body could do, what it looked like mattered less. Though her body insecurities sometimes rear their heads, they fall away as soon as she drops into her pleasure. "I can go totally into self-criticism, but generally, I've shifted how I feel about my body to be less about the external, what it looks like, and more about, 'man, our bodies are capable of so much,'" she says. "I feel happy in my body. I'm connected to my truth and my intuition."

The Highly Orgasmic Woman

Stories like these once made me jealous. Around my twenty-ninth birthday, I ended a three-year relationship with the first partner to bring me to orgasm. I was scared nobody else would. What if it was not my own body but his magic touch that enabled my orgasmicity? What if my pleasure was in his hands? I had no clue what women meant when they described full-body orgasms, multiple orgasms, or out-of-this-world, mind-blowing sex. Sex was fun but not transcendent, and masturbation was a humdrum operation.

That was when my path intersected with Sophie's. I met her on a retreat in 2019, and after hearing her story, I told her I wanted to feel how she did: receptive, alive, and orgasmic in the broadest sense of the word. Soon after, I hired her as a coach. Following our initial phone call, she gave me two woo-woo-sounding exercises: a breast self-massage and a "honey pot" meditation, where I visualized honey being poured over my clitoris, vagina, cervix, and ovaries, caressing me from the inside. After my first meditation on the unfurnished floor of my new LA apartment, I felt a diffuse wave of pleasure wash over my pelvis, leaving me refreshed and energized. As I strolled down the Venice Beach boardwalk that evening, I wondered if strangers who passed me could feel how pleasantly turned on yet somehow satiated I felt. Massaging my breasts was more triggering. Since they'd been touched and commented on without consent, involving them in sex felt objectifying. It took months of practice to tune out the internalized male gaze that had obstructed my pleasure. Once I could put those thoughts aside and touch my body just for me, I realized non-genital pleasure was key to increasing my orgasmic ability. As a protective mechanism, I'd tuned out sensations everywhere but my clitoris, creating a narrow path to pleasure. But now, my whole body was opening up.

Soon after, I met Josefina, a spiritual psychologist known as the "pussy priestess." Josefina spoke to me about laying the foundation for great sex and radiant health through self-care. She taught me to add sensual delights to my day, like drinking cacao in the morning and breathing into muscles that felt tight. When I first heard her describe herself as a highly orgasmic woman, I feared this term would never fit me. Yet deep down, I knew it was precisely what I was. I began studying to become a sex educator and therapist myself, and during my training, I learned orgasmic yoga – a practice that combines stretching, breathwork, vocalizations, dance, and self-pleasure to expand sexual sensation. Over a few months of self-massage, mindful masturbation, sexual meditations, orgasmic yoga, and daily self-care practices, I recovered the expansive sexuality that was mine all along. Orgasm was no longer a sensation I forced out of myself but one that flowed naturally from the pleasure I felt all over my body. I began orgasming through nipple stimulation, erotic dreams, and even hypnosis.

I started sleeping with someone new the next winter, and to my surprise, my mind no longer sounded like a broken record of "will I orgasm?" It was a given that I would – usually, two or three times. Unplagued by performance anxiety, I entered the bedroom with a playful curiosity about what I could feel. The nagging sense that my male partner was sexually superior and I had to "keep up" was gone. I was not putting my sexual response to the test but reveling in it. I was not a challenge or a puzzle, no – my pleasure was an honor to witness and be a part of. Never again would I settle for partners who didn't participate in it wholeheartedly. It wasn't until a few years later that I experienced my first orgasms through penetration. They happened after I started slowing down and blocking out time to just lie on the beach. I felt the sun on my skin as if *it* were penetrating my pores. I stopped working late at night and took time to relax in the bath. And soon, I began feeling so turned on and receptive that penetrative orgasms were accessible.[12] My body was no longer in fight-or-flight, so it reallocated its resources to pleasure. As I said, an orgasm is the body's way of saying "yes." To open up my orgasmic potential, I had to create a life my body could say "yes" to.

I Am Blessed

All these experiences boiled down to one change: I affirmed the pleasure I was capable of. The pleasure I was already feeling. I reveled in my sensuousness. I pictured my pelvis brimming with juicy receptors, if not actual honey. I felt my blanket nuzzling me like a lover as I lay in bed. I felt each molecule of air massaging my skin as I strolled down the street, basking in the bliss it created. Instead of clamming up or worrying sexual partners were getting bored, I laid back and imagined how exciting it must be to interface with the ball of yumminess and moans I was. I pictured my body melting into their touch, getting lost in my breath and vocalizations. This helped me orgasm with every partner I had, from a kind new acquaintance at a sex party to a Tinder match I grew to love. The common factor in these scenarios, after all, was me. Paradise lived within my body.

At times, it felt like I really was in the midst of one long orgasm that paused after sex or self-pleasure and picked back up the next time I started. Other times, it didn't even pause. It continued as I swirled my hips in dance class or lay in the savasana yoga pose while a gong played and the vibrations rippled through me. As Josefina said, life is one giant orgasm. She taught me we have the power to cultivate that pleasure by choosing where we place our focus. So, I learned to focus on what was right with my body, not what was wrong. And for the times when that became challenging, she and I created a mantra: "I am physically blessed. I am spiritually blessed. I am blessed."

Dancing Pleasurably with Pain

I'd like to say that was my happy ever after, but then 2020 happened and – oh no – 2021. And my progress seemed to fly out the window. Multiple health setbacks smacked me over the head including Covid, several adverse medication reactions, and what I later learned was mold illness. I couldn't sleep, my muscles were involuntarily twitching, my left leg periodically went numb, and when I thought it couldn't get worse, it began hurting when I touched my clitoris (see chapter 2 – mold can increase risk for yeast infections).[13] I felt, dare I say it, cursed.

On top of that, I struggled through a string of bad luck in my love life. In April 2021, after meeting someone for the first time since quarantine, I found myself at a new agey LA party. We gathered in a circle at the beginning and each announced what we hoped for from the night. I, being me, declared I'd like "the best orgasm of my life." Instead, I wandered the house looking for the guy I'd started seeing – then found him with another woman. I kept it together long enough to find a friend who was an embodiment coach. She took me out onto the patio and told me to let out my emotions. Soon, I was stomping, screaming, and sobbing in frustration over what the past year brought me – until my screams and sobs turned into shrieks and giggles. "That was like an emotional orgasm," I told her once I'd gotten it all out. My wish had been granted. Living orgasmically was not all about pleasure. Sometimes it meant leaning into pain.

That didn't mean dwelling on the pain. I climbed up from rock bottom step by step. I went back to the basics. I took walks on the beach and visited the spa just to swim mini laps in the jacuzzi. I found a functional medicine nurse who took my complaints seriously but didn't overwhelm me with expensive tests or supplements. I made my treatment plan enjoyable when possible, incorporating ayurveda, acupuncture, delicious and nutritious foods, and practitioners I could really talk to. I added pleasure to my life however I could. But sometimes that wasn't accessible, and when all I could do was sit in my bathtub and cry, I did that. I developed a fuller understanding of how I'd been looking to feel when I first spoke with Sophie. My quest for an orgasmic life wasn't really about orgasms. It was about receptivity, embodiment, and connection. And when I realized that, I realized I need not always be in a state of pleasure. It was more about feeling what was there. As Amber Hartnell told me of orgasmic birth: "If we learn how to be with our pain and stay present with it, pain actually moves and dissolves. It's not static; it's fluid, and it guides us into something deeper." Slowly, by letting that pain exist and addressing it when I could, I made the way for pleasure once more.

Later that year, I began feeling like myself again. My life was orgasmic in a different way. I wasn't feeling sexual all the time.

It had been almost two years since I'd even had sex. And yet I found myself looking forward to the littlest things: walking into my apartment with its pink and blue hues, petting my cats, sleeping on my squishy mattress pad. I was excited to be in my body. Much of the time, I still am. I may fall back into another pit of despair. Then I'll come out again, capable of feeling more deeply. As my ability to hold sorrow expands, so does my joy. And I still believe, more than ever before, that my ultimate destination is paradise. Why? Because my body has the building blocks for it. Because every woman's – every person's – does. But to unlock the blessings within our bodies, we must first see the curse we're currently under as its own type of blessing.

Tending the Garden of Eden

Throughout this book, I've charted many people's paths from pain to pleasure. I wish I could chart yours. But those I spoke to all had their own paths, lots of them brand new and some barely paved. I can't tell you which to travel, except to say it will be no one else's. What I can offer are encouraging words to cheer you on as you walk, and soothing ones to lift you when you stumble. No matter where you are on this expedition, you need not carry the baggage of blame. And while your road may be your own, your plight is not. If you struggle to feel pleasure or free yourself from pain, you are neither alone nor the problem. If it seems like suffering comes with the territory of womanhood – or just a few lucky women enjoy pleasure – that's not because we are wired for pain. Me, Josefina, and Sophie didn't have to correct any innate deficiencies. What we needed was information. My hope is that this book informs you so your journey is not as long or involved as mine. Consider it an apple in your own tree of knowledge, one you'll be rewarded for eating. And just to plant the seeds, I'll leave you with some broad advice to return you to the paradise you belong in.

1. You are the one who gets to say how much discomfort you will and won't accept. There is no amount of pain that is too small to warrant attention. Find a healthcare team invested in identifying the roots of and solutions to your problems, even if they're "normal" problems like period pain or PMS. If your doctor implies you must live with your symptoms, consult another. If you're stuck, connect with others with similar experiences. Find communities online or in person. Be patient with your body; walk your path at your own pace. But don't fall into the trap of believing where you are is where you'll stay.

2. Slow down enough to appreciate the impact of the stressors and traumas, big and little, you've endured. The emotional, the physical, and the many hurts that contain elements of both. You may not know what direction to walk in, what person to listen to, what pill to take or not take. What you know is what wounds need tending, and that will lead you toward the answers you seek. Give yourself space and time to process your pain. Talk to others you trust, professionals or friends. Write or make art. Put on music and dance. Take aimless walks with no goal other than to feel your feelings. And once in a while, take a healing break from healing. Put your health goals aside to just live.

3. Your body contains the blueprints for pleasure. The trick is living in it, not outside it. The sensations you're longing to feel are there – you need to tune in to them and trust them. Start outside the bedroom. Find sensuality in showers, walks, and meals. Attend to your five senses. Be mindful of what you see, hear, feel, smell, and taste. These sensations may not always be pleasant, but it's by sitting with discomfort that you'll expand your capacity for joy. When you feel pleasure, get excited

about it. Express it. Don't wonder if it should be bigger or different. Conceptualize your life as one big orgasm, and see what changes.

Above all, don't condemn your body or yourself. There is no apple you could eat, no wrong turn you could take, that would make you a match for your sorrow. Pain is not the price we pay for being born in our bodies. A woman's body is a gift. All bodies are. Unlimited access to pleasure is our uncorrupted state, and we get closer to this state each time we release judgment for where we are. And uplift others our paths intersect with.

Women's Bodies, Rewritten

From the philosophers of ancient Greece to the politicians of twenty-first-century America, people have professed opinions on what being female means for millennia. But there's no singular truth about women's bodies. They can be prisons of pain and numbness. They can be holders of trauma and oppression. They can be vehicles for ecstasy and rapture. They can be endless wells of orgasms. It's our choice which version of women we want filling our world. But if there's less of the former and more of the latter, we'll all be better for it. Once we've eaten from the tree of knowledge of good, women's joy comes to seem like second nature. Once we've attuned to our bodies and ourselves, we realize we were made not for suffering but for bliss. As sex-positive preacher Lyvonne Briggs so beautifully told me in the last interview I'll quote from:

> There's no scripture that says "woman, thou shalt orgasm," but when I look at the divine intelligence that's embedded in women's bodies and bearers of a clitoris, I think about how

the clitoris has one job – and it is not to procreate. It is not to defecate. It is not to urinate. It is to have all those thousands of nerve endings burst into one miraculous juicy delicious eighteen-second shiver-me-timber and shiver-up-and-down-my-spine orgasm.

Our design is kind and generous. Our capacity for joy is endless. And if that doesn't match what we see around us now, that should be a wake-up call. Our pain and pleasurelessness are not natural states but windows into problems. Not just problems plaguing individual lives, but the most momentous problems shaping all our lives. Men suffer for the lack of attention to health concerns that affect them too. For the stressful and isolated lifestyles that are imposed on them as well. For the gender essentialism that confines them just as much. For the one-sided sexual scripts that thwart their drive toward connection. For the exploitive values that affect their relationships with people and the planet. And for the suffering of those they interact with every day. We all thrive when women and sex and gender-diverse people experience the best of what their bodies have to offer. When those around us are physically and mentally healthy, our relationships become more harmonious. When our children are birthed in uplifting environments, our families are happier. When our partners are sexually free, this invites us to explore our own expansive sexuality.

Unwinding Eve's curse unwinds Adam's and everybody's in between. Once we unveil the mythology around women's pain and pleasurelessness and demand better lives for ourselves, we pave a way back to paradise for everyone. We realize our oppression is not our identity, our punishment is not our destiny. Eden was our home all along. We are physically blessed. We are spiritually blessed. We are blessed.

Epilogue: Original Virtue

Just to thank you for making it to the end, I'll tell you one more story. It was the night I met Ayelet from chapters 7 and 13, at a New Year's party carrying us into 2024. I was thirty-three and had been struggling with respiratory issues from mold. But this night brought some levity to my year. At the event in California, we'd taken a mood-elevating herb called kanna. That would be our apple for the evening, giving knowledge, giving life.

Me, Ayelet, and her husband gathered in a circle and spoke about a concept from our childhoods: repentance. They reminded me of my first encounters with a punishing God. On the "day of atonement," Yom Kippur, I'd go to temple to reflect upon the past year's wrongdoings and request God's forgiveness. I imagined God as a domineering father who scolded me for my missteps. I had to implore him to welcome me back into his arms when I had earned his disapproval. Yom Kippur is the last of ten "days of repentance" in Jewish tradition. Ayelet's husband explained the Hebrew word for repentance: *teshuvah*.

"Many Jews – and Christians – think we need God to forgive our sins, but the real translation of 'teshuvah' is 'coming back to the self,'" he said. "We don't need to be forgiven. We're already in good standing in God's eyes."

"So, it's more like a purification?" I asked.

"Not exactly," said Ayelet. "There's nothing to purify. You're already pure. All you have to do is remember who you are."

My eyes brightened as it sunk in: We weren't born with the curse of original sin. We were born with the blessing of original virtue. We needed not plead guilty, but to see our innocence. We needed not to repent for our darkness but to embrace our light. That was what Judaism was about – and Christianity too: Our "sins" have already been paid for. There is no punishment. No fall. Paradise was never really lost. As we bring Eve back to her origins, we can bring the creeds around her back to theirs. We can return people and their theology to their purity. We can come back to ourselves, a teshuvah for all humankind. All that Eve and her descendants ever needed was a grand-scale teshuvah. Not to overcome our bodies but to come back to them. To live in them. To know them. Our bodies, our souls, our societies have always already been pure. All we must do is come back to ourselves, and one another.

For the rest of the event, I lay on a mattress on the floor with another guest, Simon. I told him about this book, which I was just beginning, and posed the question: "If it's not normal or natural for women to suffer, why are so many of us suffering?"

"Who says," he asked, "that women's suffering is not normal or natural?"

"I do," I laughed. "I'm writing a whole book about it. About how women were not made to be in pain. Do you disagree?"

I held my breath as I anticipated him telling me my entire book was trash. Instead, his reply circuitously strengthened my thesis: "It is completely normal and natural to suffer when you are not being revered." *Revered*. The word rang and reverberated through my mind's ear. It was a word that had frequented my thoughts before in moments of anger, when I felt unseen or belittled. That rage was in my body. It was in every woman's body. The rage of being gazed upon and treated with irreverence. That rage of not being revered had stiffened my body, weakened my bones, haunted my brain, interrupted my sleep for so long.

This was why we had an epidemic of female pain and pleasurelessness. It was simple: We were not being revered. Women's pain and pleasurelessness were not myths. They were real. They were valid responses to relationships, homes, and communities where we were not revered. Our period cramps, painful sex, sorrowful childbirth, chronic illness, elusive orgasms, mood swings – these were our bodies' rebellions against a world that didn't revere us. Every month, every day, we were feeling what was wrong and right with the world. And there had been so much wrong. But today, there was a lot right.

"If we are revered ..." I wondered aloud. Yet the rest of the sentence was longer and vaster than words could encapsulate. It was in my body. And beyond it, with all the people in the room. And outside it. I breathed in, and the breath filled my diaphragm. Really filled it. I marveled that for the first time since my run-in with mold, my lungs could fully inhale. Tiny fasciculations in my facial muscles opened my airway. I looked around me, surveying the scene. Simon was lying to my right, gently stroking my hair. Another man I'd been talking to lay to my left, massaging my shoulder where it hurt. Shimmering trees outside reached toward the windows to caress us, their hands full of Christmas lights. And over by the fireplace was Ayelet, who had given me permission to let go of past shame. Who'd let me know that I had nothing to atone for.

"It's almost midnight," the host announced. On a whim, I turned to Simon and asked, "Would you kiss me when the clock strikes twelve?"[1]

He laughed. "Just a quick kiss. Trust me, I'd like more, but I'd want us to be fully sober for that."

We counted down to one. He turned to me. "You still want a kiss?" he asked, as if my mind could've changed in those few seconds, since last year.

I smiled and nodded my head. He inched toward me so slowly I could track his every motion, then gave me one kiss. I leaned back in for one more. I could barely hear the room's festive cheers, I was so lost in the sparkly sensation. "That's all for now," he grinned. I lay back down, taking in the starlight on the insides of my eyelids.

He got up, and I started, suddenly pulled out of the moment. "I'm going to the bathroom, but I'll be back in one minute," he reassured me. "And I'll lie right back here with you. Please don't worry."

"Why does it turn me on when you say that?" I laughed.

"Because you trust me," he smiled. "I'll be right back."

I was safe here. I breathed in. I returned the air to my lungs and remembered something I'd read: the Greek word for "breath," *pneuma*, also meant "spirit." I remembered how God breathed into Adam to bring him to life.[2] I felt free to come to life. I could feel the breath move me, shake me, traveling down to my pelvis, caressing it from the inside. I laughed and squealed; it felt kind of like … an orgasm. This was my orgasmic rebirth. I exhaled as the air answered for me: "If we are revered … then this." It was not the kind of reverence that kneeled below a pedestal. It was the kind that gave me open space. Space to breathe. I recalled something Betty Dodson told me in one of her workshops: "Orgasm lives on the breath." I was coming back to my breath, to myself. There was no trying, no striving, no altering or compensating. No repentance. Just me and some people who embraced me with arms as wide or tight as I needed. Who made room for me to take in spirit.

I let the air, the spirit, fill my limbs and move me. I danced to the other side of the room. My arms and legs roamed free from all false deities who'd condemned me. I'd eaten from the tree of knowledge, and for that, I was rewarded.

Resource List

For Sexual, Reproductive, and Pelvic Health
Pelvic Health and Rehabilitation Center: pelvicpainrehab.com
Chronic UTI Australia: chronicutiaustralia.org.au
Endometriosis Association: endometriosisassn.org
The Lady's Handbook for Her Mysterious Illness by Sarah Ramey
Ask Me About My Uterus by Abby Norman
When Sex Hurts by Andrew Goldstein, Caroline Pukall, and Irwin Goldstein
Vulvodynia, Vaginismus, & Vestibulodynia by Stephanie Prendergast, Jandra Mueller, and Elizabeth Akincilar
Living PCOS Free by Nitu Bajekal and Rohini Bajekal
You Are Not Broken podcast: kellycaspersonmd.com/you-are-not-broken-podcast
Bodies podcast: www.bodiespodcast.com
Do You Endo: doyouendo.com
Learn Body Literacy: learnbodyliteracy.com
Clue blog: helloclue.com/articles
Flo Living: floliving.com
The Egg Whisperer: draimee.org
VuvaTech: vuvatech.com

Flex: flexfits.com
Private Packs: privatepacks.com
Planned Parenthood chat line: plannedparenthood.org/online-tools/chat
Go Ask Alice: goaskalice.columbia.edu
Scarleteen: scarleteen.com
Our Bodies, Ourselves: ourbodiesourselves.org

For Help Living Orgasmically
American Association of Sexuality Educators, Counselors, and Therapists directory: aasect.org/referral-directory
Association of Certified Sexological Bodyworkers directory: sexologicalbodyworkers.org/practitioners
Becoming Cliterate by Laurie Mintz
The Ultimate Guide to Sex Over Fifty by Joan Price
My book *Subjectified: Becoming a Sexual Subject*
Coaching with me: suzannahweiss.com/sex-coaching
Josefina Bashout: josefinabashout.com
Sophie Lua: sophielua.com
My free course, The Orgasm Cure: bit.ly/orgasmcure
My courses: suzannahweiss.com/courses
Vanessa Marin's Finishing School: vmtherapy.com/finishing-school
Orgasmic Yoga: orgasmicyoga.com
Bodysex: dodsonandross.com
OMG YES: omgyes.com

For Trauma and Mental Health
The Rape, Abuse & Incest National Network: rainn.org
Crisis Text Line: 741741
Trauma Therapist Network: traumatherapistnetwork.com
CPTSD Foundation: cptsdfoundation.org
National Eating Disorders Association: www.nationaleatingdisorders.org/get-help
Neurodynamic Breathwork: breathworkonline.com

The Body Keeps the Score by Bessel van der Kolk
My Grandmother's Hands by Resmaa Menakem
In an Unspoken Voice by Peter Levine
The Borderline Personality Disorder Survival Guide by Alex L. Chapman and Kim L. Gratz
No Bad Parts by Richard Schwartz
Recovery of Your Inner Child by Lucia Capacchione
Life Without Ed by Jenni Schaefer and Thom Rutledge
The Healing You Can Do by Meghan Hindi

For Childbirth Support
DONA doula directory: dona.org/what-is-a-doula-2/find-a-doula
Pregnancy, Childbirth, and the Newborn by Penny Simkin, Janet Whalley, Ann Keppler, Janelle Durham, and April Bolding
The Birth Partner by Penny Simkin
Ina May's Guide to Childbirth by Ina May Gaskin
When Survivors Give Birth by Penny Simkin and Phyllis Klaus
The Ultimate Guide to Sex Through Pregnancy and Motherhood by Madison Young
Orgasmic Birth by Elizabeth Davis and Debra Pascali-Bonaro
Orgasmic Birth documentary: orgasmicbirth.com
Orgasmic Birth courses and coaching: orgasmicbirth.com/for-parents
Ecstatic Birth courses and coaching: ecstatic-birth.com/programs
Orgasmic Birth podcast: orgasmicbirth.com/podcast
My Pleasure and Childbirth course: bit.ly/pleasureandchildbirth
Postpartum Support International Hotline: 1-800-944-4773
National Maternal Mental Health Hotline: 1-833-852-6262

For Sensuality and Spirituality
Sensual Faith by Lyvonne Briggs

Who Told You That You Were Naked? Meditations on the Sexual Body by Beverly Dale
Red Lip Theology by Candice Marie Benbow
Bad Theology Kills by Kevin Garcia
Sensual Faith podcast: bit.ly/sensualfaithpodcast

For Learning About – and From – My Interviewees
Sophia Wallace: sophiawallace.art
Kaytlin Bailey: kaytlinbailey.com
Joan Price: joanprice.com
Hida Viloria: hidaviloria.com
Sarah Ramey: sarahmarieramey.com
Kuya'karanuta'ni Gonzalez: atabeysrisingtides.com
Ngozi Tibbs: journeylightercoaching.com
Meghan Hindi: wildishway.com
Amber Hartnell: amberhartnell.com
Meg Calvin: megcalvin.com
Celia Bedelia: x.com/_celia_bedelia_
Shanéa Thomas: instagram.com/drkchocolatnoir
Ayelet Polonsky: instagram.com/themanifestationmindset

Notes

Introduction
1. Ju, H., Jones, M., & Mishra, G. (2013). The prevalence and risk factors of dysmenorrhea. *Epidemiologic Reviews*.
2. Mitchell, K., Geary, R., Graham, C., Datta, J., Wellings, K., Sonnenberg, P., Field, N., Nunns, D., Bancroft, J., Jones, K., Johnson, A., & Mercer, C. (2017). Painful sex (dyspareunia) in women: prevalence and associated factors in a British population probability survey. *BJOG: An International Journal of Obstetrics & Gynaecology*.
3. Lloyd, E. (2006). *The Case of the Female Orgasm*. Harvard University Press.
4. Malmusi, D., Artazcoz, L., Benach, J., & Borrell, C. (2011). Perception or real illness? How chronic conditions contribute to gender inequalities in self-rated health. *The European Journal of Public Health*; Osborne, N. R. & Davis, K. D. (2022). Sex and gender differences in pain. *International Review of Neurobiology*; Remes, O., Brayne, C., van der Linde, R., & Lafortune, L. (2016). A systematic review of reviews on the prevalence of anxiety disorders in adult populations. *Brain and Behavior*; Albert, P. (2015). Why is depression more prevalent in women? *Journal of Psychiatry & Neuroscience*.

Part I The Fall
1. Waller-Bridge, P. (Writer) & Bradbeer, H. (Director). (2019). Season 2, episode 3. *Fleabag*. Two Brothers Pictures.

2. Ramey, S. (2021). *The Lady's Handbook for Her Mysterious Illness*. Anchor Books.

Chapter 1 Curses Were Meant to Be Broken

1. *Holy Bible: New International Version*. (2011). Genesis 3:16–17. Biblica.
2. Ryan, C. & Jethá, C. (2011). *Sex at Dawn*. Harper. This paragraph also draws from an email exchange with Ryan.
3. Lerner, G. (1986). *The Creation of Patriarchy*. Oxford University Press.
4. Alesina, A. F., Giuliano, P., & Nunn, N. (2011). On the origins of gender roles: Women and the plough. *SSRN Electronic Journal*.
5. Ryan & Jethá, see n. 2.
6. I'm evoking the image of an apple because it's part of modern folklore, but the word in the Bible just means "fruit" and was unlikely to describe an apple. Taylor, A. P. (2021). Was the "forbidden fruit" in the Garden of Eden really an apple? *Live Science*.
7. Gottlieb, A. (2020). Menstrual taboos: Moving beyond the curse. In C. Bobel (ed.), *The Palgrave Handbook of Critical Menstruation Studies*. Palgrave Macmillan.
8. Abbas, K., Usman, G., Ahmed, M., Qazi, R., Asghar, A., Masood Shah, A., Rizvi, A., Abid, K., Haq, K. U., Tahir, A., & Usama, S. M. (2020). Physical and psychological symptoms associated with premenstrual syndrome and their impact on the daily routine of women in a low socioeconomic status locality. *Cureus*; Bureau, T. H. (2023). Close to 12% of young girls think menstruation is a curse from God or caused by disease: study. *The Hindu*.
9. De Palma, B. (Director) & Cohen, L. D. (Writer). (1976). *Carrie*. Red Bank Films.
10. Joffe, N. F. (1948). The vernacular of menstruation. *WORD*; Larsen, V. L. (1963). Psychological study of colloquial menstrual expressions. *Northwest Medicine*.
11. Lee, J. (1994). Menarche and the (hetero) sexualization of the female body. *Gender and Society*.
12. Meriwether, E., Rosenstock, K., Addelman, R. (Writers), & Woliner, J. (Director). (2012). *New Girl*. "Menzies." Season 2, episode 7. Elizabeth Meriwether Pictures.
13. MacMillan, C. (2023). Endometriosis is more than just "painful periods." yalemedicine.org.

14. Bougie, O., Nwosu, I., & Warshafsky, C. (2022). Revisiting the impact of race/ethnicity in endometriosis. *Reproduction and Fertility*; Endometriosis Foundation of America (2020). The endometriosis resource portal for people of color. endofound.org.
15. Ju, Jones, & Mishra, see Introduction, n. 1.
16. Dusenbery, M. (2019). *Doing Harm*. HarperOne.
17. American College of Obstetricians and Gynecologists (2020). Dysmenorrhea: Painful periods. acog.org.
18. Iacovides, S., Avidon, I., & Baker, F. C. (2015). What we know about primary dysmenorrhea today: A critical review. *Human Reproduction Update*.
19. Cleveland Clinic (2022). Prostaglandins. my.clevelandclinic.org. King, S. (2024). Black box: The reduction and mystification of the menstrual cycle in western school and medical education. In K. Standing, S. Parker, & S. Lotter (eds.), *Experiences of Menstruation from the Global South and North*. Oxford University Press.
20. Coco, A. S. (1999). Primary dysmenorrhea. *American Family Physician*; Chan, W. Y. & Hill, J. C. (1978). Determination of menstrual prostaglandin levels in non-dysmenorrheic and dysmenorrheic subjects. *Prostaglandins*; Sacco, K., Portelli, M., Pollacco, J., Schembri-Wismayer, P., & Calleja-Agius, J. (2011). The role of prostaglandin E2 in endometriosis. *Gynecological Endocrinology*; Chan, W. Y., Dawood, M. Y., & Fuchs, F. (1981). Prostaglandins in primary dysmenorrhea. *The American Journal of Medicine*.
21. McKenna, K. A. & Fogleman, C. D. (2021). Dysmenorrhea. *American Family Physician*.
22. World Health Organization (2016). Dioxins and their effects on human health. who.int.
23. Bruner-Tran, K., Ding, T., & Osteen, K. (2010). Dioxin and endometrial progesterone resistance. *Seminars in Reproductive Medicine*; Rier, S. (1993). Endometriosis in rhesus monkeys (Macaca mulatta) following chronic exposure to 2,3,7,8-tetrachlorodibenzo-p-dioxin. *Fundamental and Applied Toxicology*.
24. Newer bleaching methods have reduced dioxin levels in menstrual products, but there are still trace amounts, which have an impact when exposed to absorbent vaginal tissue over time. Dudley, S., Nassar, S., Hartman, E., & Wang, S. (2017). Tampon safety. National Center for Health Research. center4research.org; Campaign for Safe Cosmetics (2024). Menstrual care products and toxic chemicals.

safecosmetics.org; Marroquin, J., Kiomourtzoglou, M. A., Scranton, A., & Pollack, A. Z. (2023). Chemicals in menstrual products: A systematic review. *BJOG: An International Journal of Obstetrics and Gynaecology*; World Health Organization (2016). Dioxins and their effects on human health. who.int.
25. Women in Balance Institute (2012). Xenoestrogens: What are they, how to avoid them. womeninbalance.org.
26. Marroquin et al., see n. 24.
27. Maghrifi, D. S., Lestari, P., & Sa'adi, A. (2022). View of association between food plastic packaging and dysmenorrhea in female adolescents. *Journal of Maternal and Child Health*.
28. Dutta, S., Banu, S. K., & Arosh, J. A. (2023). Endocrine disruptors and endometriosis. *Reproductive Toxicology*.
29. European Commission (2014). Consumers: Commission improves safety of cosmetics. ec.europa.eu; Milman, O. (2019). US cosmetics are full of chemicals banned by Europe – why? *The Guardian*.
30. Barnard, N. (2000). Diet and sex-hormone binding globulin, dysmenorrhea, and premenstrual symptoms. *Obstetrics & Gynecology*.
31. Najafi, N., Khalkhali, H., Moghaddam Tabrizi, F., & Zarrin, R. (2018). Major dietary patterns in relation to menstrual pain: A nested case control study. *BMC Women's Health*.
32. Fernández-Martínez, E., Onieva-Zafra, M. D., & Parra-Fernández, M. L. (2018). Lifestyle and prevalence of dysmenorrhea among Spanish female university students. *PLOS ONE*.
33. North American Menopause Society (2022). What you eat could contribute to your menstrual cramps. menopause.org.
34. LaMotte, S. (2022). You can fight menstrual cramps with food, studies say. *CNN*.
35. Rahbar, N., Asgharzadeh, N., & Ghorbani, R. (2012). Effect of omega-3 fatty acids on intensity of primary dysmenorrhea. *International Journal of Gynecology & Obstetrics*.
36. Tempels, T., Verweij, M., & Blok, V. (2017). Big Food's ambivalence: Seeking profit and responsibility for health. *American Journal of Public Health*.
37. Onieva-Zafra, M. D., Fernández-Martínez, E., Abreu-Sánchez, A., Iglesias-López, M. T., García-Padilla, F. M., Pedregal-González, M., & Parra-Fernández, M. L. (2020). Relationship between diet, menstrual pain and other menstrual characteristics among Spanish students. *Nutrients*; Deutch, B. (1995). Menstrual pain in Danish

women correlated with low n-3 polyunsaturated fatty acid intake. *European Journal of Clinical Nutrition*; Naraoka, Y., Hosokawa, M., Minato-Inokawa, S., & Sato, Y. (2023). Severity of menstrual pain is associated with nutritional intake and lifestyle habits. *Healthcare*.

38. Finance Watch (2019). Financialisation of food. finance-watch.org; World Wildlife Fund (2024). Sustainable agriculture. worldwildlife.org; Anomaly, J. (2014). What's wrong with factory farming? *Public Health Ethics*.

39. Arsenault, C. (2014). Only 60 years of farming left if soil degradation continues. *Scientific American*; Bretveld, R. W., Thomas, C. M., Scheepers, P. T., Zielhuis, G. A., & Roeleveld, N. (2006). Pesticide exposure: The hormonal function of the female reproductive system disrupted? *Reproductive Biology and Endocrinology*; Mnif, W., Hassine, A. I., Bouaziz, A., Bartegi, A., Thomas, O., & Roig, B. (2011). Effect of endocrine disruptor pesticides: A review. *International Journal of Environmental Research and Public Health*; Provenza, F. D., Kronberg, S. L., & Gregorini, P. (2019). Is grassfed meat and dairy better for human and environmental health? *Frontiers in Nutrition*.

40. Cassata, C. (2019). How stress can cause a hormonal imbalance. *Healthline*.

41. Triwahyuningsih, R. Y., Rahfiludin, M. Z., Sulistiyani, S., & Widjanarko, B. (2024). Role of stress and physical activity on primary dysmenorrhea: A cross-sectional study. *Narra J*; Matsumura, K., Tsuno, K., Okamoto, M., Takahashi, A., Kurokawa, A., Watanabe, Y., & Yoshida, H. (2023). The association between the severity of dysmenorrhea and psychological distress of women working in central Tokyo – A preliminary study. *International Journal of Environmental Research and Public Health*; László, K. D., Győrffy, Z., Ádám, S., Csoboth, C., & Kopp, M. S. (2008). Work-related stress factors and menstrual pain: A nation-wide representative survey. *Journal of Psychosomatic Obstetrics & Gynecology*.

42. Wang, L. (2004). Stress and dysmenorrhoea: A population based prospective study. *Occupational and Environmental Medicine*.

43. Jeong, D.-K., Lee, H. K., & Kim, J. (2023). Effects of sleep pattern, duration, and quality on premenstrual syndrome and primary dysmenorrhea in Korean high school girls. *BMC Women's Health*; Armour, M., Ee, C. C., Naidoo, D., Ayati, Z., Chalmers, K. J., Steel,

K. A., de Manincor, M. J., & Delshad, E. (2019). Exercise for dysmenorrhoea. *Cochrane Database of Systematic Reviews.*
44. For an in-depth discussion of the politics of what counts as "real" medicine, see Ramey, Part 1, n. 2.
45. Bible Gateway (2015). Leviticus 20:18. biblegateway.com.
46. Mazokopakis, E. E. & Samonis, G. (2018). Is vaginal sexual intercourse permitted during menstruation? A biblical (Christian) and medical approach. *Mædica.*
47. Some Christians believe Jesus' crucifixion already undid the curse. As retired bishop Roya King tells me: "The work on the cross of Jesus Christ ended the Edenic curses. We're free and don't even know to what extent we really are."
48. *Holy Bible: New International Version.* (2011). Genesis 3:14–17. Biblica.
49. Latthe, P., Latthe, M., Say, L., Gülmezoglu, M., & Khan, K. S. (2006). WHO systematic review of prevalence of chronic pelvic pain: A neglected reproductive health morbidity. *BMC Public Health.*
50. World Health Organization (2023). Endometriosis. who.int; Zimmermann, A., Bernuit, D., Gerlinger, C., Schaefers, M., & Geppert, K. (2012). Prevalence, symptoms and management of uterine fibroids: An international internet-based survey of 21,746 women. *BMC Women's Health*; Deswal, R., Narwal, V., Dang, A., & Pundir, C. S. (2020). The prevalence of polycystic ovary syndrome: A brief systematic review. *Journal of Human Reproductive Sciences.*
51. Iacovides, S., Avidon, I., & Baker, F. C. (2015). What we know about primary dysmenorrhea today: A critical review. *Human Reproduction Update.*
52. Britton, C. J. (1996). Learning about "the curse": An anthropological perspective on experiences of menstruation. *Women's Studies International Forum.*

Chapter 2 Women's Natural Defectiveness and Other Greek Myths

1. Wray, A. A., Velasquez, J., & Khetarpal, S. (2020). Balanitis. StatPearls; Cleveland Clinic (2023). Balanitis. my.clevelandclinic.org; McMillen, M. (2015). Balanitis: A penis condition explained. WebMD.
2. Aristotle (1912). *The Works of Aristotle, Volume V.* Trans. J. A. Smith & W. D. Ross. Clarendon Press.

3. Aristotle (2020). *The History of Animals*. Trans. D'Arcy Wentworth Thompson; Collins Dictionary (2024). Pubes. collinsdictionary.com.
4. I'm referencing two different translations here. The first quote comes from J. A. Smith and W. D. Ross. The second comes from *The Second Sex* by Simone de Beauvoir. While de Beauvoir doesn't cite a source, she appears to be translating a statement from *On the Generation of Animals*, which Smith and Ross translate as "we must look upon the female character as being a sort of natural deficiency." Aristotle, see n. 2; de Beauvoir, S. (2011). *The Second Sex*. Knopf Doubleday.
5. Laqueur, T. (1990). *Making Sex*. Harvard University Press.
6. Cobb, M. (2008). *Generation: The Seventeenth-Century Scientists Who Unraveled the Secrets of Sex, Life, and Growth*. Bloomsbury.
7. Magee, J. (2020). Women. Thomistic Philosophy Page. aquinasonline.com.
8. Baskin, L., Shen, J., Sinclair, A., Cao, M., Liu, X., Liu, G., Isaacson, D., Overland, M., Li, Y., & Cunha, G. R. (2018). Development of the human penis and clitoris. *Differentiation*; Aatsha, P. A., Arbor, T. C., & Krishan, K. (2020). Embryology, sexual development. StatPearls.
9. Park, K. (1997). The rediscovery of the clitoris. In C. Mazzio and D. Hillman (eds.), *The Body in Parts: Fantasies of Corporeality in Early Modern Europe*. Routledge.
10. Weiss, S. (2017). "Fear of the clit": A brief history of medical books erasing women's genitalia. *Vice*.
11. O'Connell, H. E., Sanjeevan, K. V., & Hutson, J. M. (2005). Anatomy of the clitoris. *Journal of Urology*; Gross, R. E. (2022). Half the world has a clitoris. Why don't doctors study it? *The New York Times*.
12. Weiss, S. (2019). The insidious reasons doctors are botching labiaplasties. *The Establishment*.
13. Cleveland Clinic, see n. 1; Brazier, Y. (2024). What to know about balanitis. *Medical News Today*.
14. Pauls, R. N. (2015). Anatomy of the clitoris and the female sexual response. *Clinical Anatomy*. Pauls confirmed with me via email that these measurements come from cadaver studies and MRI studies in unaroused states, so the clitoris is likely larger when engorged.
15. It might appear, then, that the clitoris is *bigger* than the penis – but there's an internal portion of the penis too, with a "bulb" and "crura" similar to the clitoris. Still, the clitoris is closer in size to the penis

than believed. Weiss, S. (2024). Your penis is bigger than you might think. *Men's Health*.
16. Baskin et al., see n. 8.
17. National Library of Medicine (2024). Clitoris. meshb.nlm.nih.gov; National Library of Medicine (2024). Penis. meshb.nlm.nih.gov.
18. Orenstein, P. (2017). What young women believe about their own sexual pleasure. TED.
19. UNESCO (2018). International technical guidance on sexuality education: An evidence-informed approach. unfpa.org.
20. Geller, S. E., Adams, M. G., & Carnes, M. (2006). Adherence to federal guidelines for reporting of sex and race/ethnicity in clinical trials. *Journal of Women's Health*; Geller, S. E., Koch, A., Pellettieri, B., & Carnes, M. (2011). Inclusion, analysis, and reporting of sex and race/ethnicity in clinical trials: Have we made progress? *Journal of Women's Health*.
21. Beery, A. K. & Zucker, I. (2011). Sex bias in neuroscience and biomedical research. *Neuroscience & Biobehavioral Reviews*.
22. Dusenbery, see chapter 1, n. 16.
23. Windgassen, S. S., Sutherland, S., Finn, M. T. M., Bonnet, K. R., Schlundt, D. G., Reynolds, W. S., Dmochowski, R. R., & McKernan, L. C. (2022). Gender differences in the experience of interstitial cystitis/bladder pain syndrome. *Frontiers in Pain Research*; Weiss, S. (2019). What causes interstitial cystitis? How 10 women got to the root of their bladder pain. *Bustle*; Chung, M. K., Chung, R. R., Gordon, D., & Jennings, C. (2002). The evil twins of chronic pelvic pain syndrome: endometriosis and interstitial cystitis. *Journal of the Society of Laparoendoscopic Surgeons*.
24. Johns Hopkins Medicine (2024). Interstitial cystitis. hopkinsmedicine.org; Mayo Clinic (2024). Interstitial cystitis. mayoclinic.org.
25. Weiss, S. (2019). "I've gained my life back": New tests may help those with persistent urinary tract infections. *The Washington Post*.
26. Little, P., Turner, S., Rumsby, K., Jones, R., Warner, G., Moore, M., Lowes, J. A., Smith, H., Hawke, C., Leydon, G., & Mullee, M. (2010). Validating the prediction of lower urinary tract infection in primary care: Sensitivity and specificity of urinary dipsticks and clinical scores in women. *British Journal of General Practice*.
27. Heytens, S., Sutter, A. D., Coorevits, L., Cools, P., Boelens, J., Simaey, L. V., Christiaens, T., Vaneechoutte, M., & Claeys, G. (2017). Women with symptoms of a urinary tract infection but a negative

urine culture: PCR-based quantification of Escherichia coli suggests infection in most cases. *Clinical Microbiology and Infection.*
28. Wojno, K. J., Baunoch, D., Luke, N., Opel, M., Korman, H., Kelly, C., Jafri, S. M. A., Keating, P., Hazelton, D., Hindu, S., Makhloouf, B., Wenzler, D., Sabry, M., Burks, F., Penaranda, M., Smith, D. E., Korman, A., & Sirls, L. (2020). Multiplex PCR based urinary tract infection (UTI) analysis compared to traditional urine culture in identifying significant pathogens in symptomatic patients. *Urology.*
29. Shute, N. (2013). Common test for bladder infections misses too many cases. *NPR.*
30. Heytens et al., see n. 27.
31. Yang, X., Chen, H., Zheng, Y., Qu, S., Wang, H., & Yi, F. (2022). Disease burden and long-term trends of urinary tract infections: A worldwide report. *Frontiers in Public Health.*
32. There's some confusion over how to define IC. Were America and I misdiagnosed, since our symptoms stemmed from an infection? The thing is, many cases diagnosed as IC seem to stem from chronic low-grade infections. The definition itself is fuzzy, as IC is a syndrome – a condition characterized by symptoms rather than etiology. Whatever we call it, what's important is not assuming it will always be lifelong. Bono, M. J., Reygaert, W. C., & Leslie, S. W. (2023). Urinary tract infection. StatPearls.
33. Chronic UTI Australia (2023). Hearing patient voices: Capturing the impacts of chronic urinary tract infection. chronicutiaustralia.org.

Chapter 3 From Stained Sheets to White Houses: The Painful Price of Pleasure

1. I'm curious, however, if there are other interpretations, as the passage doesn't explicitly mention blood. *Holy Bible: New International Version.* (2011). Deuteronomy 22:17. Biblica.
2. Koller, A. (2010). Sex or power? The crime of the bride in Deuteronomy 22. *Journal for Ancient Near Eastern and Biblical Law.* This paragraph is also based on a conversation with Koller.
3. Harris, K. & Caskey-Sigety, L. (2014). *The Medieval Vagina.* CreateSpace Independent Publishing Platform; Lemay, H. R. (1992). *Women's Secrets: A Translation of Pseudo-Albertus Magnus' De Secretis Mulierum with Commentaries.* SUNY Press; Blank, H. (2008). *Virgin: The Untouched History.* Bloomsbury USA.

4. Beaumont-Thomas, B. (2019). Outrage as US rapper TI says he has daughter's hymen checked annually. *The Guardian*.
5. World Health Organization (2018). Eliminating virginity testing: An interagency statement. iris.who.int.
6. Heath, N. (2018). The historic tradition of wedding night-virginity testing. *SBS*.
7. Carlton, V. (2004). "White Houses." On *Harmonium*. A&M Records.
8. This interviewee chose not to use her real name, so "Amanda" will be her pseudonym.
9. Online Etymology Dictionary (2024). Hymen. etymonline.com.
10. Maugh, T. H. (2009). Swedes say it is no longer a hymen – it's a vaginal corona. *Los Angeles Times*.
11. Paterson-Brown, S. (1998). Commentary: Education about the hymen is needed. *British Medical Journal*; Nazaralieva, A., Bocharova, M., & Nyurkina, S. (2023). Frequency of bleeding at first vaginal intercourse and stereotypes surrounding it: A pilot survey of 7426 Russian-speaking women. 24th World Meeting on Sexual Medicine; Adams, J. A., Botash, A. S., & Kellogg, N. (2004). Differences in hymenal morphology between adolescent girls with and without a history of consensual sexual intercourse. *Archives of Pediatrics & Adolescent Medicine*.
12. Curtis, E. & Lazaro, C. S. (1999). Appearance of the hymen in adolescents is not well documented. *British Medical Journal*.
13. Emans, S. J., Woods, E. R., Allred, E. N., & Grace, E. (1994). Hymenal findings in adolescent women: Impact of tampon use and consensual sexual activity. *Journal of Pediatrics*.
14. There are also some girls born without hymens, though this is rare. Hegazy, A. A. & Al-Rukban, M. O. (2012). Hymen: Facts and conceptions. *TheHealth*; Schaffir, J. (2020). The hymen's tale: Myths and facts about the hymen. Ohio State University; Jenny, C., Kuhns, M. L., & Arakawa, F. (1987). Hymens in newborn female infants. *Pediatrics*.
15. Joannides, P. (2022). *The Guide to Getting It On*. Goofy Foot Press; Mishori, R., Ferdowsian, H., Naimer, K., Volpellier, M., & McHale, T. (2019). The little tissue that couldn't – dispelling myths about the hymen's role in determining sexual history and assault. *Reproductive Health*; McCann, J., Miyamoto, S., Boyle, C., & Rogers, K. (2007). Healing of hymenal injuries in prepubertal and adolescent girls: A descriptive study. *Pediatrics*.

16. Cleveland Clinic (2022). Septate hymen. my.clevelandclinic.org; Cleveland Clinic (2022). Imperforate hymen. my.clevelandclinic.org.
17. Gunter, J. (2019). *The Vagina Bible*. Kensington.
18. Cleveland Clinic (2022). Hymen. my.clevelandclinic.org.
19. Konaç, A. (2024). A 7-year retrospective analysis of hymenoplasty: Profiles from a specialized gynecological cosmetic surgery practice. *Aesthetic Surgery Journal*; Saraiya, H. A. (2015). Surgical revirgination: Four vaginal mucosal flaps for reconstruction of a hymen. *Indian Journal of Plastic Surgery*; Prakash, V. & Garg, N. (2016). Revirgination is not the same as hymenoplasty. *PMFA News*.
20. Herrmann, B., Banaschak, S., Csorba, R., Navratil, F., & Dettmeyer, R. (2014). Physical examination in child sexual abuse. *Deutsches Aerzteblatt*; Salazar, A. A. C. (1976). Notes on the virgo intacto. *Cenipec Revista*; Mykhailychenko, B., Biliakov, M., & Ergard, A. (2000). Practical trainings from forensic medicine. UkrDGRI Publishing House; Merriam-Webster Dictionary (2024). Virgo intacta. Merriam-Webster.com.
21. Bailey, A. (2015). The limits of physical evidence in sex abuse cases. *Global Health News*; Adams, J. A., Harper, K., Knudson, S., & Revilla, J. (2024). Examination findings in legally confirmed child sexual abuse: It's normal to be normal. *Pediatrics*.
22. Mishori et al., see n. 15; Hegazy & Al-Rukban, see n. 14.
23. Torres-Cueco, R. & Nohales-Alfonso, F. (2021). Vulvodynia – it is time to accept a new understanding from a neurobiological perspective. *International Journal of Environmental Research and Public Health*; Faye, R. B. & Piraccini, E. (2020). Vulvodynia. StatPearls; Johns Hopkins Medicine (2024). Endometriosis. hopkinsmedicine.org; see chapter 2, n. 24.
24. Bornstein, J., Goldstein, A. T., Stockdale, C. K., Bergeron, S., Pukall, C., Zolnoun, D., & Coady, D. (2016). 2015 ISSVD, ISSWSH and IPPS consensus terminology and classification of persistent vulvar pain and vulvodynia. *Obstetrics & Gynecology*.
25. Those with all three conditions are over five times more likely than those without any of them to have vulvodynia. Reed, B. D., Harlow, S. D., Sen, A., Edwards, R. M., Chen, D., & Haefner, H. K. (2012). Relationship between vulvodynia and chronic comorbid pain conditions. *Obstetrics & Gynecology*.
26. For an in-depth discussion about the language we use to describe

sex and how it shortchanges women, see my first book: Weiss, S. (2024). *Subjectified*. Polity.
27. Mayo Clinic (2024). Painful intercourse (dyspareunia). mayoclinic.org.
28. Nygaard, I. (2008). Prevalence of symptomatic pelvic floor disorders in US women. *JAMA*.
29. Abraham, C. (2020). Experiencing vaginal dryness? Here's what you need to know. American College of Obstetricians and Gynecologists. acog.org.
30. Kingsberg, S. A., Wysocki, S., Magnus, L., & Krychman, M. L. (2013). Vulvar and vaginal atrophy in postmenopausal women: Findings from the REVIVE (REal Women's VIews of Treatment Options for Menopausal Vaginal ChangEs) Survey. *Journal of Sexual Medicine*.
31. Bonafide (2021). The state of menopause. hellobonafide.com.
32. Google Dictionary (2024). Normal.
33. Price, J. (2015). *The Ultimate Guide to Sex after 50*. Cleis Press.
34. The original Hebrew passage has also been translated as "I will greatly increase your painful conception." *Holy Bible: King James Version* (2017). Genesis 3:16. Green World Classics; Dijk-Coombes, V. & Marian, R. (2020). Towards a new understanding of the curse of Eve: Female sexual pain in Genesis 3:16 and other ancient texts. *Scriptura*; Kadari, T. (2009). Eve: Midrash and Aggadah. *Shalvi/Hyman Encyclopedia of Jewish Women*. jwa.org.

Chapter 4 Men's Bodies Are from Mars, Women's Are from Venus

1. "S/he," pronounced "she," is a pronoun used by some intersex people.
2. An ectopic pregnancy is one where the fertilized egg is someplace outside the uterus, such as in the fallopian tube.
3. This number is debated as it includes a wide variety of physiological traits considered sex-atypical. The number of people with genitalia that doctors consider ambiguous is estimated at around .05%. Blackless, M., Charuvastra, A., Derryck, A., Fausto-Sterling, A., Lauzanne, K., & Lee, E. (2000). How sexually dimorphic are we? Review and synthesis. *American Journal of Human Biology*; Intersex Society of North America (2008). How common is intersex? isna.org.
4. Laqueur, see chapter 2, n. 5.
5. Fausto-Sterling, A. (1992). *Myths Of Gender: Biological Theories About Women and Men*. Basic Books.

6. Silverman, D. L. (1992). *Art Nouveau in Fin-de-Siècle France: Politics, Psychology, and Style.* University of California Press.
7. Quinlan, S. M. (2021). *Morbid Undercurrents: Medical Subcultures in Postrevolutionary France.* Cornell University Press.
8. Laqueur, see chapter 2, n. 5.
9. Gray, J. (2012). *Men Are from Mars, Women Are from Venus.* Harper Paperbacks.
10. Langhorne, O., Thomas, K., & Standeven, L. (2024). How sex changes after menopause. Johns Hopkins Medicine. hopkinsmedicine.org; Cappelletti, M. & Wallen, K. (2016). Increasing women's sexual desire: The comparative effectiveness of estrogens and androgens. *Hormones and Behavior*; Kelly, A. M., Gonzalez Abreu, J. A., & Thompson, R. R. (2022). Beyond sex and aggression: Testosterone rapidly matches behavioural responses to social context and tries to predict the future. *Proceedings of the Royal Society B: Biological Sciences.* The last study cited here is a rodent study, but I'm also drawing upon references 9–10 in this paper, which are human studies.
11. "Borikua" and "Boricua" are Indigenous terms for people from the island most Americans know as Puerto Rico. Because Puerto Rico was named by Spanish colonizers, these terms help Indigenous people reclaim their own identity, according to Kuya.
12. Brogan, M. K. (2022). For centuries, Two-Spirit people had to carry out Native traditions in secret. Now, they're "making their own history." *VCU News*; Lyons, M. (2015). How European settlers destroyed two-spirit tradition. *Xtra.*
13. Josi, T. and Picq, M. (2019). Indigenous sexualities: Resisting conquest and translation. In C. Cottet and M. L. Picq (eds.), *Sexuality and Translation in World Politics.* E-International Relations; Brekus, C. A. (2017). Women and religion in colonial North America and the United States. *Oxford Research Encyclopedia of American History.* oxfordre.com.
14. Warren, C. A. (2014). Gender reassignment surgery in the 18th century: A case study. *Sexualities.*
15. InterAct (2021). Intersex definitions. interactadvocates.org.
16. Griffiths, D. A. (2018). Diagnosing sex: Intersex surgery and "sex change" in Britain 1930–1955. *Sexualities.*
17. Human Rights Watch (2017). "I want to be like nature made me": Medically unnecessary surgeries on intersex children in the US. hrw.org.

18. Goymann, W., Brumm, H., & Kappeler, P. M. (2022). Biological sex is binary, even though there is a rainbow of sex roles. *BioEssays*.
19. Ainsworth, C. (2015). Sex redefined. *Nature*.
20. Foreman, M., Hare, L., York, K., Balakrishnan, K., Sánchez, F. J., Harte, F., Erasmus, J., Vilain, E., & Harley, V. R. (2018). Genetic link between gender dysphoria and sex hormone signaling. *Journal of Clinical Endocrinology & Metabolism*.
21. Independent Lens (2015). Interactive map: Gender-diverse cultures. *PBS*.
22. American Psychiatric Association (2017–). Gender dysphoria diagnosis. psychiatry.org.
23. Nirappil, F. (2023). For trans people, medical visits can be more traumatizing than healing. *The Washington Post*.
24. National Center for Transgender Equality (2015). The Report of the US Transgender Survey. transequality.org.
25. UNAIDS (2022). 20.2 million girls and women living with HIV. unaids.org.
26. Bradley, E. L. P., Williams, A. M., Green, S., Lima, A. C., Geter, A., Chesson, H. W., & McCree, D. H. (2019). Disparities in incidence of human immunodeficiency virus infection among black and white women – United States, 2010–2016. *Morbidity and Mortality Weekly Report*.
27. Ruschak, I., Montesó-Curto, P., Rosselló, L., Aguilar Martín, C., Sánchez-Montesó, L., & Toussaint, L. (2023). Fibromyalgia syndrome pain in men and women: A scoping review. *Healthcare*; Arora, H. C. & Shoskes, D. A. (2015). The enigma of men with interstitial cystitis/bladder pain syndrome. *Translational Andrology and Urology*.
28. Rei, C., Williams, T., & Feloney, M. (2018). Endometriosis in a man as a rare source of abdominal pain: A case report and review of the literature. *Case Reports in Obstetrics and Gynecology*.
29. Harvard Health Blog (2016). Understanding the heart attack gender gap. health.harvard.edu; European Society of Cardiology (2023). Women more likely to die after heart attack than men. escardio.org; O'Connor, A. (2022). Why heart disease in women is so often missed or dismissed. *The New York Times*.
30. Joel, D., Berman, Z., Tavor, I., Wexler, N., Gaber, O., Stein, Y., Shefi, N., Pool, J., Urchs, S., Margulies, D. S., Liem, F., Hänggi, J., Jäncke, L., & Assaf, Y. (2015). Sex beyond the genitalia: The human brain mosaic. *Proceedings of the National Academy of Sciences*.

Chapter 5 How the Female Orgasm Became Elusive

1. Ephron, N. (Writer) & Reiner, R. (Director). (1989). *When Harry Met Sally.* Castle Rock Entertainment; Star, D., Rottenberg, J., & Zuritsky, E. (Writers) & Engler, M. (Director). (2001). *Sex and the City.* Season 4, episode 8. HBO; David, L., Seinfeld, J., & Levy, L. H. (Writers) & Cherones, T. (Director). (1993). *Seinfeld.* Season 5, episode 1. Castle Rock Entertainment.
2. Thatcher, A. (2016). *Redeeming Gender.* Oxford University Press.
3. Aristotle, the Famous Philosopher (2010). *Aristotle's Masterpiece.* The Ex-classics Project.
4. Though the two-sex model was starting to take hold at this point, the one-sex model did not completely vanish, nor did knowledge of the clitoris. Laqueur, see chapter 2, n. 5.
5. The Decameron Web (2011). Sexual desire. Brown University. brown.edu.
6. Ehrenreich, B. and English, D. (2010). *Witches, Midwives, and Nurses: A History of Women Healers.* The Feminist Press at CUNY.
7. Laqueur, see chapter 2, n. 5.
8. Laqueur, see chapter 2, n. 5; Trouille, M. S. (1997). *Sexual Politics in the Enlightenment: Women Writers Read Rousseau.*
9. Proctor, C. E. (1990). *Women, Equality, and the French Revolution.* Praeger.
10. Cott, N. F. (1978). Passionlessness: An interpretation of Victorian sexual ideology, 1790–1850. *Signs.*
11. Gregory, J. (1808). *A Father's Legacy to his Daughters.* T. Cadell and W. Davies.
12. Cott, see n. 10; Smith, A. (2003). Not an Indian tradition: The sexual colonization of Native peoples. *Hypatia*; Croisy, S. (2017). Fighting colonial violence in "Indian Country": Deconstructing racist sexual stereotypes of Native American Women in American popular culture and history. *Angles.*
13. Acton, W. (2023). *The Functions and Disorders of the Reproductive Organs.* Legare Street Press.
14. Blechner, M. (2017). The clitoris: Anatomical and psychological issues. *Studies in Gender and Sexuality.*
15. Van de Velde, T. H. (1955). *Ideal Marriage: Its Physiology and Technique.* William Heinemann Medical Books; Goodreads (2024). Ideal Marriage, Its Physiology and Technique. goodreads.com.
16. Stains, L. R. & Bechte, S. (1996). *Sex: A Man's Guide.* Rodale.

17. Kerner, I. (2004). *She Comes First: The Thinking Man's Guide to Pleasuring a Woman*. William Morrow.
18. Solot, D. & Miller, M. (2007). *I Love Female Orgasm*. Marlowe and Company.
19. "You will never see (that I'm aware of) a movie scene in a late-night comedy where a woman, overcome with desire, accidentally comes too fast," the article reads. Indeed, this doesn't happen in the movies, but it happens in real life. In a Portuguese study of 510 women, 58% reported orgasming sooner than they wished at least once in a while. Moore, T. (2013). Are you sure you want an orgasm EVERY time? *Jezebel*; Carvalho, S., Moreira, A., Rosado, M., Correia, D., Maia, D., & Pimentel, P. (2011). Female premature orgasm: Does this exist? *Sexologies*.
20. Hochman, A. (2022). Pleasure quest: In search of the elusive orgasm. WebMD; Scutti, S. (2016). The ancient evolutionary origin of the elusive female orgasm. *CNN*.
21. Herbenick, D., Reece, M., Schick, V., Sanders, S. A., Dodge, B., & Fortenberry, J. D. (2010). An event-level analysis of the sexual characteristics and composition among adults ages 18 to 59: Results from a national probability sample in the United States. *Journal of Sexual Medicine*.
22. Andrejek, N., Fetner, T., & Heath, M. (2022). Climax as work: Heteronormativity, gender labor, and the gender gap in orgasms. *Gender & Society*; Rissel, C., Badcock, P. B., Smith, A. M. A., Richters, J., de Visser, R. O., Grulich, A. E., & Simpson, J. M. (2014). Heterosexual experience and recent heterosexual encounters among Australian adults: The Second Australian Study of Health and Relationships. *Sexual Health*; Kontula, O. (2015). Sex life challenges: The Finnish case. In J. D. Wright (ed.), *International Encyclopedia of the Social & Behavioral Sciences*. Elsevier; Beauchamp, Z. (2014). 6 maps and charts that explain sex around the world. *Vox*.
23. Brizendine, L. (2007). *The Female Brain*. Harmony.
24. Zietsch, B. P. & Santtila, P. (2013). No direct relationship between human female orgasm rate and number of offspring. *Animal Behaviour*; see Introduction, n. 3.
25. The information provided on peristalsis draws from an email exchange with Robert King, Professor of Applied Psychology at University College Cork. The Baker & Bellis (1993) study Brizendine cites doesn't prove her claim, as it found women's orgasms assisted

with sperm transport if they occurred *anywhere* between a minute before and forty-five minutes after ejaculation – and its results failed to replicate. Towne, J. P. & Gallup, G. G. (2016). Female copulatory orgasm. In T. K. Shackelford & V. A. Weekes-Shackelford (eds.), *Encyclopedia of Evolutionary Psychological Science*. Springer; Zervomanolakis, I., Ott, H. W., Hadziomerovic, D., Mattle, V., Seeber, B. E., Virgolini, I., Heute, D., Kissler, S., Leyendecker, G., & Wildt, L. (2007). Physiology of upward transport in the human female genital tract. *Annals of the New York Academy of Sciences*; King, R., Dempsey, M., & Valentine, K. A. (2016). Measuring sperm backflow following female orgasm: A new method. *Socioaffective Neuroscience & Psychology*; King, R. (2024). *Naturally Selective: Evolution, Orgasm, and Female Choice*. CRC Press; Baker, R. R. & Bellis, M. A. (1993). Human sperm competition: Ejaculate manipulation by females and a function for the female orgasm. *Animal Behaviour*.

26. Thomashauer, R. (2018). *Pussy: A Reclamation*. Hay House.
27. Kinsey, A. (1998). *Sexual Behavior in the Human Female*. Indiana University Press.
28. The researchers shared the median measure since it's less affected by extreme outliers than the mean. I'm also aware of recent studies showing figures like thirteen and fourteen minutes to orgasm during partnered sex. The study producing the thirteen-minute figure had questionable methodology, with women timing themselves starting when they became "adequately aroused" – so it's unclear if they were receiving clitoral stimulation (or any stimulation) the whole time. In the survey finding fourteen minutes (twelve for those without orgasmic difficulties), it's also unclear what was taking place in these women's encounters. Either way, this research reflects women's current circumstances more than their potential. Until we have sexual equality, data will reflect the inequalities that exist. That said, enjoying a long buildup to orgasm is not a bad thing – in fact, the data likely includes women who extend it intentionally. For Goodness Sake (2018). Second OMGYES pleasure report [unpublished data set]; Bhat, G. S. & Shastry, A. (2020). Time to orgasm in women in a monogamous stable heterosexual relationship. *Journal of Sexual Medicine*; Rowland, D. L., Sullivan, S. L., Hevesi, K., & Hevesi, B. (2018). Orgasmic latency and related parameters in women during partnered and masturbatory sex. *Journal of Sexual Medicine*.

29. There is a line in Kinsey's *Sexual Behavior in the Human Female* stating that a woman "may need 10 or 20 minutes or more to reach [orgasm] in coitus," which may be the real source of this figure – but it appears to be a general observation rather than an empirical finding. Weiss, S. (2018). What a fake "female orgasm" statistic says about gender bias. *The Establishment*; Weiten, W., Dunn, D. S., & Yost Hammer, E. (2011). *Psychology Applied to Modern Life*. Cengage Learning; see n. 27.
30. The claim that female orgasm requires trust and relaxation is also invalidating to those who climax unwillingly during assaults. See n. 23; Mount Sinai Adolescent Health Center (2019). You asked it: Do victims sometimes orgasm during sexual assault? teenhealthcare.org.
31. Wise, N. J., Frangos, E., & Komisaruk, B. R. (2017). Brain activity unique to orgasm in women: An fMRI analysis. *Journal of Sexual Medicine*.
32. See chapter 8 for research on how rape culture impacts women's sexual response.
33. Richters, J., de Visser, R., Rissel, C., & Smith, A. (2006). Sexual practices at last heterosexual encounter and occurrence of orgasm in a national survey. *Journal of Sex Research*; Armstrong, E. A., England, P., and Fogarty, A. C. K. (2009). Orgasm in college hookups and relationships. In B. Risman (ed.), *Families as They Really Are*. W. W. Norton.
34. Hite, S. (1976). *The Hite Report*. Macmillan.
35. See Introduction, n. 3.
36. Frederick, D. A., St. John, H. K., Garcia, J. R., & Lloyd, E. A. (2017). Differences in orgasm frequency between gay, lesbian, bisexual, and heterosexual men and women in a US national sample. *Archives of Sexual Behavior*.
37. Google Dictionary (2024). Sex, Sexual intercourse.
38. Herbenick, D., Bowling, J., Fu, T.-C., Dodge, B., Guerra-Reyes, L., & Sanders, S. (2017). Sexual diversity in the United States: Results from a nationally representative probability sample of adult women and men. *PLOS ONE*; Wood, J. R., McKay, A., Komarnicky, T., & Milhausen, R. R. (2016). Was it good for you too?: An analysis of gender differences in oral sex practices and pleasure ratings among heterosexual Canadian university students. *The Canadian Journal of Human Sexuality*; Andrejek, Fetner, & Heath, see n. 22.
39. Volck, W., Ventress, Z. A., Herbenick, D., Adams Hillard, P. J., &

Huppert, J. S. (2013). Gynecologic knowledge is low in college men and women. *Journal of Pediatric and Adolescent Gynecology*.
40. Google Dictionary (2024). Foreplay.
41. See n. 34.
42. See n. 34.
43. RB (2016). K-Y® Intense® is giving women a reason to fake it no more. *PR Newswire*; Foria (2024). Awaken arousal oil with CBD. foriawellness.com.
44. Matlock, D. (2024). G-Shot. drmatlock.com. Stats on the number of doctors offering the procedure and the price are from a search on realself.com.
45. Thompson, H. (2018). G-spot surgery given to three women to boost sexual pleasure. *New Scientist*.
46. The Maerks Institute (2024). G-Spot enhancement. themaercks institute.com. I'm also drawing from a PR pitch I received via email from this business, which boasts: "This eliminates the need for pillows under the buttocks during intercourse."
47. The Orgasmatron has fallen off the radar since then. Canner, E. (Director). (2009). *Orgasm Inc*. Astrea Media; Dawson, B. (2021). Who killed the "female pleasure button"? *MEL*.
48. O-Shot (2024). O-Shot® Official Home Page. oshot.info.
49. Luxury Listings NYC (2017). Sexual revolution. calameo.com.
50. It's common for people to prefer touch on the clitoral hood over direct touch on the glans. Some articles reference a "hooded clitoris," claiming too big a hood impedes pleasure, but "hooded clitoris" is not a medical term except insofar as plastic surgeons promote their services with it.
51. Dodson, B. (2009). Hate being a woman because it's so hard to orgasm. dodsonandross.com.
52. See n. 34.

Chapter 6 PMS, from "a Raging Animal" to "Blood Coming Out of Her Wherever"

1. American College of Obstetricians and Gynecologists (2024). Premenstrual syndrome. acog.org.
2. Sattar, K. (2014). Epidemiology of premenstrual syndrome – a systematic review and meta-analysis study. *Journal of Clinical and Diagnostic Research*; National Health Service (2024). PMS (premenstrual syndrome). nhs.uk.

3. Harvard Health Blog (2017). Premenstrual dysphoria disorder: It's biology, not a behavior choice. health.harvard.edu; El Gamal, E. (2023). Premenstrual syndrome (PMS) and premenstrual dysphoric disorder (PMDD). American Psychiatric Association. psychiatry.org.
4. Johnson, T. M. (1987). Premenstrual syndrome as a western culture-specific disorder. *Culture, Medicine and Psychiatry*.
5. Ussher, J. M. & Perz, J. (2011). PMS as a gendered illness linked to the construction and relational experience of hetero-femininity. *Sex Roles*.
6. LA Times Archives (1987). Dr. Edgar Berman at 72: Author, aide, chauvinist. *Los Angeles Times*.
7. Ironside, A. (2008). Marc Rudov on "the downside" of a woman president: "You mean besides the PMS and the mood swings, right?" *Media Matters*.
8. Mosbergen, D. (2015). Female CEO says women "shouldn't be president" because of "different hormones," "biblical reasoning." *The Huffington Post*.
9. CNN (2015). Donald Trump: I don't respect Megyn Kelly (CNN interview with Don Lemon). youtube.com.
10. Weisz, G. & Knaapen, L. (2009). Diagnosing and treating premenstrual syndrome in five western nations. *Social Science & Medicine*; Chrysler, J. & Caplan, P. (2002). The strange case of Dr. Jekyll and Ms. Hyde: How PMS became a cultural phenomenon and a psychiatric disorder. *Annual Review of Sex Research*.
11. Shorter, E. (2005). *A Historical Dictionary of Psychiatry*. Oxford University Press.
12. Chrysler & Caplan, see n. 10; Brozan, N. (1982). Premenstrual syndrome: A complex issue. *The New York Times*; New York Times Archives (1981). British legal debate: Premenstrual tension and criminal behavior. *The New York Times*.
13. Cosgrove, L. & Riddle, B. (2003). Constructions of femininity and experiences of menstrual distress. *Women & Health*.
14. It's not that estrogen and progesterone don't impact mood; low estrogen can exacerbate PMS and PMDD, says King. But there's no evidence that it's the root cause. King, see chapter 1, n. 19.
15. Chrysler & Caplan, see n. 10.
16. Marvan, Ma. L. & Escobedo, C. (1999). Premenstrual symptomatology. *Psychosomatic Medicine*; Cosgrove & Riddle, see n. 13.

17. Ramjohn, R. (Host). (2019). PMS is real. PMS isn't real. [Podcast episode]. *Hormonal*.
18. Siminiuc, R. & Țurcanu, D. (2023). Impact of nutritional diet therapy on premenstrual syndrome. *Frontiers in Nutrition*; Hashim, M. S., Obaideen, A. A., Jahrami, H. A., Radwan, H., Hamad, H. J., Owais, A. A., Alardah, L. G., Qiblawi, S., Al-Yateem, N., & Faris, M. A.-I. E. (2019). Premenstrual syndrome is associated with dietary and lifestyle behaviors among university students: A cross-sectional study from Sharjah, UAE. *Nutrients*; Latif, S., Naz, S., Ashraf, S., & Ahmed Jafri, S. (2022). Junk food consumption in relation to menstrual abnormalities among adolescent girls: A comparative cross sectional study. *Pakistan Journal of Medical Sciences*.
19. Park, J., Lee, J. J., Park, S., Lee, H., Nam, S., Lee, S., & Lee, H. (2022). Endocrine disrupting chemicals and premenstrual syndrome in female college students in East Asia: A multi-country study. *International Journal of Women's Health*; Yesildere Saglam, H. & Orsal, O. (2020). Effect of exercise on premenstrual symptoms: A systematic review. *Complementary Therapies in Medicine*; Triebner, K., Markevych, I., Bertelsen, R. J., Sved Skottvoll, B., Hustad, S., Forsberg, B., Franklin, K. A., Holm, M., Lindberg, E., Heinrich, J., Gómez Real, F., & Dadvand, P. (2022). Lifelong exposure to residential greenspace and the premenstrual syndrome: A population-based study of Northern European women. *Environment International*.
20. Mishra, S. & Marwaha, R. (2023). Premenstrual dysphoric disorder. StatPearls.
21. De Carvalho, A. B., Cardoso, T. A., Mondin, T. C., Da Silva, R. A., Souza, L. D., Magalhães, P. V., & Jansen, K. (2018). Prevalence and factors associated with premenstrual dysphoric disorder: A community sample of young adult women. *Psychiatry Research*; Skrzypulec-Plinta, V., Drosdzol, A., Nowosielski, K., & Plinta, R. (2010). The complexity of premenstrual dysphoric disorder – risk factors in the population of Polish women. *Reproductive Biology and Endocrinology*; Maity, S., Wray, J., Coffin, T., Nath, R., Nauhria, S., Sah, R., Waechter, R., Ramdass, P., & Nauhria, S. (2022). Academic and social impact of menstrual disturbances in female medical students: A systematic review and meta-analysis. *Frontiers in Medicine*; Ussher, J. M. & Perz, J. (2020). "I feel fat and ugly and hate myself": Self-objectification through negative constructions of premenstrual embodiment. *Feminism & Psychology*.

22. ResearchGate Blog (2016). Why do we still not know what causes PMS? researchgate.net.
23. Gillings, M. R. (2014). Were there evolutionary advantages to premenstrual syndrome? *Evolutionary Applications*; Reiber, C. (2008). An evolutionary model of premenstrual syndrome. *Medical Hypotheses*.
24. Todd, N. (2022). Slideshow: A visual guide to premenstrual syndrome (PMS). WebMD.
25. Vitti, A. (2014). *Woman Code*. HarperOne. This statement also draws from a conversation with Vitti.
26. Downie, J., Poyser, N. L., & Wunderlich, M. (1974). Levels of prostaglandins in human endometrium during the normal menstrual cycle. *Journal of Physiology*.
27. Gold, E. B., Wells, C., & Rasor, M. O. (2016). The association of inflammation with premenstrual symptoms. *Journal of Women's Health*.
28. Gurung, P., Yetiskul, E., & Jialal, I. (2019). Physiology, male reproductive system. StatPearls.
29. Murray Law, B. (2011). Hormones & desire. *Monitor on Psychology*.
30. Batrinos, M. L. (2012). Testosterone and aggressive behavior in man. *International Journal of Endocrinology & Metabolism*.
31. Ray, L. & Michalowski, M. (2022). What is the menstrual cycle? Clue. helloclue.com; Yen, J., Lin, H., Lin, P., Liu, T., Long, C., & Ko, C. (2019). Early- and late-luteal-phase estrogen and progesterone levels of women with premenstrual dysphoric disorder. *International Journal of Environmental Research and Public Health*.
32. Steinem, G. (2020). If men could menstruate. In C. Bobel, I. T. Winkler, B. Fahs, K. A. Hasson, E. A. Kissling, & T. A. Roberts (eds.), *The Palgrave Handbook of Critical Menstruation Studies*. Palgrave Macmillan.
33. Casperson, K. (Host). (2024). Myths and truths – GSM and pelvic hormones [Podcast episode]. *You Are Not Broken*.
34. Ussher, J. M. & Perz, J. (2011). PMS as a gendered illness linked to the construction and relational experience of hetero-femininity. *Sex Roles*.
35. Browne, T. K. (2014). Is premenstrual dysphoric disorder really a disorder? *Journal of Bioethical Inquiry*; see also n. 17.
36. Romans, S., Clarkson, R., Einstein, G., Petrovic, M., & Stewart, D. (2012). Mood and the menstrual cycle: A review of prospective data studies. *Gender Medicine*.

37. Potter, J., Bouyer, J., Trussell, J., & Moreau, C. (2009). Premenstrual syndrome prevalence and fluctuation over time: Results from a French population-based survey. *Journal of Women's Health.*
38. Stewart, D. E. (1989). Positive changes in the premenstrual period. *Acta Psychiatrica Scandinavica.*
39. See n. 34.
40. The American College of Obstetricians and Gynecologists recommends avoiding caffeine, minimizing fat, salt, and sugar intake, and eating complex carbs to reduce PMS symptoms. American College of Obstetricians and Gynecologists (2024). Premenstrual syndrome. acog.org.
41. Lazzaro, S. C., Rutledge, R. B., Burghart, D. R., & Glimcher, P. W. (2016). The impact of menstrual cycle phase on economic choice and rationality. *PLOS ONE.*
42. Leeners, B., Kruger, T. H. C., Geraedts, K., Tronci, E., Mancini, T., Ille, F., Egli, M., Röblitz, S., Saleh, L., Spanaus, K., Schippert, C., Zhang, Y., & Hengartner, M. P. (2017). Lack of associations between female hormone levels and visuospatial working memory, divided attention and cognitive bias across two consecutive menstrual cycles. *Frontiers in Behavioral Neuroscience.*

Chapter 7 The Institutionalization of Sorrowful Childbirth

1. Bible Hub (2024). Genesis 3:16. biblehub.com.
2. Walton doesn't believe "in sorrow thou shalt bring forth children" applies exclusively to women because he reads Eve as a symbol of companionship and community. Under this interpretation, it is everyone who reproduces anxiously.
3. Law, T. (2022). Home births became more popular during the pandemic. But many insurers still don't cover them. *Time*; United States Government Accountability Office (2023). Information on births, workforce, and midwifery education. gao.gov.
4. While not the focus of this chapter, other factors including financial interests and government policies drove the medicalization of childbirth. See Hall, L. K. (2019). *The Medicalization of Birth and Death.* Johns Hopkins University Press.
5. Forceps are plier-like instruments used to help pull a baby out. Epstein, R. H. (2011). *Get Me Out.* W. W. Norton; Newell, F. (1908). The effect of over-civilization on maternity. *The American Journal of the Medical Sciences.*

6. Thomasson, M. A. & Treber, J. (2008). From home to hospital: The evolution of childbirth in the United States, 1928–1940. *Explorations in Economic History*; National Museum of African American History & Culture (2022). The historical significance of doulas and midwives. nmaahc.si.edu; Placksin, S. (2000). *Mothering the New Mother*. William Morrow.
7. Skowronski, G. A. (2015). Pain relief in childbirth: Changing historical and feminist perspectives. *Anaesthesia and Intensive Care*.
8. Djanogly, T., Nicholls, J., Whitten, M., & Lanceley, A. (2022). Choice in episiotomy – fact or fantasy: A qualitative study of women's experiences of the consent process. *BMC Pregnancy and Childbirth*; Bohren, M. A., Mehrtash, H., Fawole, B., Maung, T. M., Balde, M. D., Maya, E., Thwin, S. S., Aderoba, A. K., Vogel, J. P., Irinyenikan, T. A., Adeyanju, A. O., Mon, N. O., Adu-Bonsaffoh, K., Landoulsi, S., Guure, C., Adanu, R., Diallo, B. A., Gülmezoglu, A. M., Soumah, A. M., & Sall, A. O. (2019). How women are treated during facility-based childbirth in four countries: A cross-sectional study with labour observations and community-based surveys. *The Lancet*.
9. Cleveland Clinic (2022). Episiotomy: Procedure, advantages, complications & healing. my.clevelandclinic.org.
10. Centers for Disease Control and Prevention (2014). Births – method of delivery. cdc.gov; World Health Organization (2021). Caesarean section rates continue to rise, amid growing inequalities in access. who.int; Althabe, F. & Belizán, J. M. (2006). Caesarean section: The paradox. *The Lancet*.
11. Deneux-Tharaux, C., Carmona, E., Bouvier-Colle, M.-H., & Bréart, G. (2006). Postpartum maternal mortality and cesarean delivery. *Obstetrics & Gynecology*; Angolile, C. M., Max, B. L., Mushemba, J., & Mashauri, H. L. (2023). Global increased cesarean section rates and public health implications: A call to action. *Health Science Reports*.
12. While those who get C-sections may have more risk factors to begin with, the study found C-sections contributed to 37% of the complications. Leonard, S. A., Main, E. K., & Carmichael, S. L. (2019). The contribution of maternal characteristics and cesarean delivery to an increasing trend of severe maternal morbidity. *BMC Pregnancy and Childbirth*.

13. Korb, D., Goffinet, F., Seco, A., Chevret, S., & Deneux-Tharaux, C. (2019). Risk of severe maternal morbidity associated with cesarean delivery and the role of maternal age: A population-based propensity score analysis. *Canadian Medical Association Journal*.
14. The COVID-19 pandemic impacted these rates, but even by 2019, the rate had almost tripled. Berg, C., Atrash, H., Koonin, L., & Tucker, M. (1996). Pregnancy-related mortality in the United States, 1987–1990. *Obstetrics & Gynecology*; Hoyert, D. (2023). Maternal mortality rates in the United States, 2021. Centers for Disease Control and Prevention. cdc.gov; Ahmad, A. (2023). America has the highest maternal mortality rate among developed nations – and it's on the rise. Here's why we are facing a pregnancy health crisis. *Fortune*.
15. Sung, S. & Mahdy, H. (2023). Cesarean section. StatPearls.
16. Liu, C., Underhill, K., Aubey, J. J., Samari, G., Allen, H. L., & Daw, J. R. (2024). Disparities in mistreatment during childbirth. *JAMA Network Open*.
17. Oelhafen, S., Trachsel, M., Monteverde, S., Raio, L., & Müller, E. C. (2021). Informal coercion during childbirth: Risk factors and prevalence estimates from a nationwide survey of women in Switzerland. *BMC Pregnancy and Childbirth*.
18. Hardin, A. M. & Buckner, E. B. (2004). Characteristics of a positive experience for women who have unmedicated childbirth. *Journal of Perinatal Education*; Hodnett, E. (2002). Pain and women's satisfaction with the experience of childbirth: A systematic review. *American Journal of Obstetrics and Gynecology*.
19. Snowden, J. M., Tilden, E. L., Snyder, J., Quigley, B., Caughey, A. B., & Cheng, Y. W. (2015). Planned out-of-hospital birth and birth outcomes. *New England Journal of Medicine*.
20. National Perinatal Epidemiology Unit (2020). The birthplace cohort study: Key findings. npeu.ox.ac.uk.
21. Çalik, K. Y., Karabulutlu, Ö., & Yavuz, C. (2018). First do no harm – interventions during labor and maternal satisfaction: A descriptive cross-sectional study. *BMC Pregnancy and Childbirth*; Lothian, J. A. (2019). Healthy birth practice #4: Avoid interventions unless they are medically necessary. *Journal of Perinatal Education*; Birthplace in England Collaborative Group (2011). Perinatal and maternal outcomes by planned place of birth for healthy women with low

risk pregnancies: The Birthplace in England National Prospective Cohort Study. *BMJ*.

22. And that's only if they've been with the company for at least a year and the company has at least fifty local employees. Forty percent of women don't qualify. US Department of Labor (2023). Fact Sheet #28: The Family and Medical Leave Act. dol.gov; Froese, M. (2023). Maternity leave in the United States: Facts you need to know. *Healthline*; Hidalgo-Padilla, L., Toyama, M., Zafra-Tanaka, J. H., Vives, A., & Diez-Canseco, F. (2023). Association between maternity leave policies and postpartum depression: A systematic review. *Archives of Women's Mental Health*; Jones, K. & Wilcher, B. (2019). Reducing maternal labor market detachment: A role for paid family leave. American Economic Association Annual Meeting; Ruhm, C. J. (2000). Parental leave and child health. *Journal of Health Economics*; Winegarden, C. R. & Bracy, P. M. (1995). Demographic consequences of maternal-leave programs in industrial countries: Evidence from fixed-effects models. *Southern Economic Journal*.

23. Placksin, see n. 6; Manning, S. S. (2018). Decolonizing birth: Women take back their power as life-givers. *Yes!*; Bachlakova, P. (2016). Indigenous doulas are reclaiming birthing practices colonization tried to erase. *Vice*.

24. Pirdel, M. & Pirdel, L. (2009). Perceived environmental stressors and pain perception during labor among primiparous and multiparous women. *Journal of Reproduction & Infertility*.

25. Goodfellow, C. F., Hull, M. G., Swaab, D. F., Dogterom, J., & Buijs, R. M. (1983). Oxytocin deficiency at delivery with epidural analgesia. *British Journal of Obstetrics and Gynaecology*; Garcia-Lausin, L., Perez-Botella, M., Duran, X., Mamblona-Vicente, M. F., Gutierrez-Martin, M. J., Gómez de Enterria-Cuesta, E., & Escuriet, R. (2019). Relation between length of exposure to epidural analgesia during labour and birth mode. *International Journal of Environmental Research and Public Health*; Antonakou, A. & Papoutsis, D. (2016). The effect of epidural analgesia on the delivery outcome of induced labour: A retrospective case series. *Obstetrics and Gynecology International*; Bakhamees, H. & Hegazy, E. (2014). Does epidural increase the incidence of cesarean delivery or instrumental labor in Saudi populations? *Middle East Journal of Anaesthesiology*; American Pregnancy Association (2024). Epidural – everything you should know about it. americanpregnancy.org.

From Cleveland Clinic: Epidural (2021), Forceps Delivery (2022), Vacuum Extraction Delivery (2022). my.clevelandclinic.org.
26. Simkin, P. & Klaus, P. (2004). *When Survivors Give Birth*. Classic Day Publishing.
27. Hendrickson, S. & Bedayn, J. (2023). More states are requiring patients to give consent for medical students performing pelvic exams. *Associated Press*.
28. Rúger-Navarrete, A., Vázquez-Lara, J. M., Antúnez-Calvente, I., Rodríguez-Díaz, L., Riesco-González, F. J., Palomo-Gómez, R., Gómez-Salgado, J., & Fernández-Carrasco, F. J. (2023). Antenatal fear of childbirth as a risk factor for a bad childbirth experience. *Healthcare*; Aksoy, H., Yücel, B., Aksoy, U., Acmaz, G., Aydin, T., & Babayigit, M. A. (2016). The relationship between expectation, experience and perception of labour pain: An observational study. *SpringerPlus*.
29. Waldenström, U., Bergman, V., & Vasell, G. (1996). The complexity of labor pain: Experiences of 278 women. *Journal of Psychosomatic Obstetrics & Gynecology*; Cheyney, M., Bovbjerg, M., Everson, C., Gordon, W., Hannibal, D., & Vedam, S. (2014). Outcomes of care for 16,924 planned home births in the United States: The Midwives Alliance of North America Statistics Project, 2004 to 2009. *Journal of Midwifery & Women's Health*.
30. Whitburn, L. Y., Jones, L. E., Davey, M.-A., & Small, R. (2017). The meaning of labour pain: How the social environment and other contextual factors shape women's experiences. *BMC Pregnancy and Childbirth*.
31. National Association of Certified Professional Midwives (2024). Legal recognition of CPMs. nacpm.org; Krebs, N. (2022). As home births rise in popularity, some midwives operate in a legal gray area. *NPR*.
32. Gregory, E., Osterman, M., & Valenzuela, C. (2022). Changes in home births by race and Hispanic origin and state of residence of mother: United States, 2019–2020 and 2020–2021. *National Vital Statistics Reports*.
33. MacDorman, M. F. & Declercq, E. (2018). Trends and state variations in out-of-hospital births in the United States, 2004–2017. *Birth*.
34. Hoyert, see n. 14.
35. HEAR HER Campaign (2024). Disparities and resilience among American Indian and Alaska Native people who are pregnant or postpartum. cdc.gov.

36. Waldman, A. (2017). How hospitals are failing black mothers. *ProPublica*.
37. American Midwifery Certification Board (2020). 2020 Demographic Report. amcbmidwife.org; Law, M. T. & Marks, M. S. (2009). Effects of occupational licensing laws on minorities: Evidence from the progressive era. *Journal of Law and Economics*; Nayak, A. (2024). The history that explains today's shortage of black midwives. *Time*.
38. Holland, B. (2018). The "father of modern gynecology" performed shocking experiments on slaves. *History*.
39. Hoffman, K. M., Trawalter, S., Axt, J. R., & Oliver, M. N. (2016). Racial bias in pain assessment and treatment recommendations, and false beliefs about biological differences between blacks and whites. *Proceedings of the National Academy of Sciences*.
40. Lathan, E. C., Britt, A., Ravi, M., Ash, M. J., McAfee, E., Wallace, S., Johnson, C., Woods-Jaeger, B., Powers, A., & Michopoulos, V. (2023). When reproduction is no longer autonomous. *Journal of Trauma & Dissociation*.
41. Klittmark, S., Malmquist, A., Karlsson, G., Ulfsdotter, A., Grundström, H., & Nieminen, K. (2023). When complications arise during birth: LBTQ people's experiences of care. *Midwifery*.
42. For this conceptualization of the female body as a cipher, I credit Ramey, see Part 1, n. 2.

Chapter 8 Trauma: An Assault on the Body
1. Taub, A. (2014). Rape culture isn't a myth. It's real, and it's dangerous. *Vox*; Rutherford, A. (2011). Sexual violence against women. *Psychology of Women Quarterly*.
2. Brownmiller, S. (1975). *Against Our Will: Men, Women and Rape*. Simon and Schuster.
3. Lazarus, M. & Wunderlich, R. (Directors). (1975). *Rape Culture*. Cambridge Documentary Films.
4. World Health Organization (2021). Devastatingly pervasive: 1 in 3 women globally experience violence. who.int.
5. Association of American Universities (2020). Report on the AAU Campus Climate Survey on Sexual Assault and Misconduct. aau.edu.
6. Jayasinghe, Y., Sasongko, V., Lim, R. K., Grover, S., Tabrizi, S. N., Moore, E. E., Donath, S., & Garland, S. M. (2017). The association between unwanted sexual experiences and early-onset cervical cancer and precancer by age 25: A case–control study. *Journal of*

Women's Health; Hindin, P., Btoush, R., & Carmody, D. P. (2019). History of childhood abuse and risk for cervical cancer among women in low-income areas. *Journal of Women's Health*.
7. Harris, H. R., Wieser, F., Vitonis, A. F., Rich-Edwards, J., Boynton-Jarrett, R., Bertone-Johnson, E. R., & Missmer, S. A. (2018). Early life abuse and risk of endometriosis. *Human Reproduction*.
8. Peters, K. M., Kalinowski, S. E., Carrico, D. J., Ibrahim, I. A., & Diokno, A. C. (2007). Fact or fiction – Is abuse prevalent in patients with interstitial cystitis? Results from a community survey and clinic population. *Journal of Urology*.
9. Seth, A. & Teichman, J. M. H. (2008). Differences in the clinical presentation of interstitial cystitis/painful bladder syndrome in patients with or without sexual abuse history. *Journal of Urology*; Karsten, M. D. A., Wekker, V., Bakker, A., Groen, H., Olff, M., Hoek, A., Laan, E. T. M., & Roseboom, T. J. (2020). Sexual function and pelvic floor activity in women: The role of traumatic events and PTSD symptoms. *European Journal of Psychotraumatology*; Dydyk, A. M. & Givler, A. (2021). Central pain syndrome. StatPearls.
10. Gardenswartz, C. (2024). Recognizing the impact of big T and little T trauma. *Psychology Today*; Ergos Institute (2024). About Dr. Levine. somaticexperiencing.com.
11. Pulverman, C. S., Kilimnik, C. D., & Meston, C. M. (2018). The impact of childhood sexual abuse on women's sexual health: A comprehensive review. *Sexual Medicine Reviews*.
12. Staples, J., Rellini, A. H., & Roberts, S. P. (2011). Avoiding experiences: Sexual dysfunction in women with a history of sexual abuse in childhood and adolescence. *Archives of Sexual Behavior*.
13. Rellini, A. H. & Clifton, J. (2011). Female orgasmic disorder. *Advances in Psychosomatic Medicine*.
14. Ehler, A., Natanagara, G., and Tuohy, K. (2019). Affirmative consent policies at the federal, state, and university levels. University of Vermont. uvm.edu; Crowe, J. & Ribeiro, G. (2024). Most states now have affirmative sexual consent laws, but not enough people know what they mean. *The Conversation*; Uhnoo, S., Erixon, S., & Bladini, M. (2024). The wave of consent-based rape laws in Europe. *International Journal of Law, Crime and Justice*.
15. Guttmacher Institute (2023). Sex and HIV education. guttmacher.org.
16. Planned Parenthood (2016). New study: Overwhelming support for consent education in schools. plannedparenthoodaction.org.

17. Margetts, J. (2015). The Line domestic violence campaign targets young attitudes towards relationships, sex. *ABC News*.
18. Tetik, S. & Yalçınkaya Alkar, Ö. (2021). Vaginismus, dyspareunia and abuse history: A systematic review and meta-analysis. *Journal of Sexual Medicine*.
19. Latimer, R. L., Vodstrcil, L. A., Fairley, C. K., Cornelisse, V. J., Chow, E. P. F., Read, T. R. H., & Bradshaw, C. S. (2018). Non-consensual condom removal, reported by patients at a sexual health clinic in Melbourne, Australia. *PLOS ONE*.
20. Baxter, A. J., Scott, K. M., Ferrari, A. J., Norman, R. E., Vos, T., & Whiteford, H. A. (2014). Challenging the myth of an "epidemic" of common mental disorders: Trends in the global prevalence of anxiety and depression between 1990 and 2010. *Depression and Anxiety*; Arnold, L. M. (2003). Gender differences in bipolar disorder. *Psychiatric Clinics of North America*; Striegel-Moore, R. H., Rosselli, F., Perrin, N., DeBar, L., Wilson, G. T., May, A., & Kraemer, H. C. (2009). Gender difference in the prevalence of eating disorder symptoms. *International Journal of Eating Disorders*.
21. Neumann, S. A. & Waldstein, S. R. (2001). Similar patterns of cardiovascular response during emotional activation as a function of affective valence and arousal and gender. *Journal of Psychosomatic Research*.
22. Weigard, A., Loviska, A. M., & Beltz, A. M. (2021). Little evidence for sex or ovarian hormone influences on affective variability. *Scientific Reports*.
23. Barrett, L. F., Robin, L., Pietromonaco, P. R., & Eyssell, K. M. (1998). Are women the "more emotional" sex? Evidence from emotional experiences in social context. *Cognition & Emotion*.
24. James, S. E., Herman, J. L., Rankin, S., Keisling, M., Mottet, L., & Anafi, M. (2016). The Report of the 2015 US Transgender Survey. National Center for Transgender Equality. transequality.org.
25. Durwood, L., McLaughlin, K. A., & Olson, K. R. (2017). Mental health and self-worth in socially transitioned transgender youth. *Journal of the American Academy of Child & Adolescent Psychiatry*.
26. Khadr, S., Clarke, V., Wellings, K., Villalta, L., Goddard, A., Welch, J., Bewley, S., Kramer, T., & Viner, R. (2018). Mental and sexual health outcomes following sexual assault in adolescents: A prospective cohort study. *The Lancet Child & Adolescent Health*.
27. Chen, L. P., Murad, M. H., Paras, M. L., Colbenson, K. M., Sattler,

A. L., Goranson, E. N., Elamin, M. B., Seime, R. J., Shinozaki, G., Prokop, L. J., & Zirakzadeh, A. (2010). Sexual abuse and lifetime diagnosis of psychiatric disorders: Systematic review and meta-analysis. *Mayo Clinic Proceedings*.
28. Mayo Clinic (2023). Chronic stress puts your health at risk. mayoclinic.org.
29. Miller, C. (2019). *Know My Name*. Viking.
30. Levenson, E. & Cooper, A. (2018). Andrea Constand's full victim impact statement about Bill Cosby's assault. *CNN*.
31. Senthilingam, M. (2017). Sexual harassment: How it stands around the globe. *CNN*; UN Women (2021). Prevalence and reporting of sexual harassment in UK public spaces. unwomenuk.org.
32. Eom, E., Restaino, S., Perkins, A. M., Neveln, N., & Harrington, J. W. (2014). Sexual harassment in middle and high school children and effects on physical and mental health. *Clinical Pediatrics*; Houle, J. N., Staff, J., Mortimer, J. T., Uggen, C., & Blackstone, A. (2011). The impact of sexual harassment on depressive symptoms during the early occupational career. *Society and Mental Health*; Magnavita, N., Di Stasio, E., Capitanelli, I., Lops, E. A., Chirico, F., & Garbarino, S. (2019). Sleep problems and workplace violence: A systematic review and meta-analysis. *Frontiers in Neuroscience*; Steine, I. M., Skogen, J. C., Hysing, M., Puigvert, L., Schønning, V., & Sivertsen, B. (2021). Sexual harassment and assault predict sleep disturbances and is partly mediated by nightmares: Findings from a national survey of all university students in Norway. *Journal of Sleep Research*.
33. Hackett, R. A., Steptoe, A., & Jackson, S. E. (2019). Sex discrimination and mental health in women: A prospective analysis. *Health Psychology*; Platt, J., Prins, S., Bates, L., & Keyes, K. (2016). Unequal depression for equal work? How the wage gap explains gendered disparities in mood disorders. *Social Science & Medicine*.
34. Wilson, E. C., Chen, Y.-H., Arayasirikul, S., Raymond, H. F., & McFarland, W. (2016). The impact of discrimination on the mental health of trans* female youth and the protective effect of parental support. *AIDS and Behavior*.
35. Runarsdottir, E., Smith, E., & Arnarsson, A. (2019). The effects of gender and family wealth on sexual abuse of adolescents. *International Journal of Environmental Research and Public Health*; Sedlak, A. J., Mettenburg, J., Basena, M., Petta, I., McPherson, K., Greene, A., &

Li, S. (2010). *Fourth National Incidence Study of Child Abuse and Neglect (NIS-4): Report to Congress.* US Department of Health and Human Services. acf.hhs.gov.

36. Ohio Alliance to End Sexual Violence (2021). Sexual violence & women of color: A fact sheet. oaesv.org; National Black Women's Justice Institute (2023). Black women, sexual assault, and criminalization. nbwji.org; National Organization for Women (2018). Black women & sexual violence. now.org.
37. Shimo, A. (2019). Are sexual abuse victims being diagnosed with a mental disorder they don't have? *The Guardian*; Gutiérrez, N. Y. (2022). The pain we carry: Healing from complex PTSD for people of color. *New Harbinger*; Kerig, P. K., Galano, M. M., & Guilaran, J. (2021). Journal of Traumatic Stress virtual special issue on complex PTSD: Classical and cutting-edge perspectives. *Journal of Traumatic Stress*.
38. Battle, C. L., Shea, M. T., Johnson, D. M., Yen, S., Zlotnick, C., Zanarini, M. C., Sanislow, C. A., Skodol, A. E., Gunderson, J. G., Grilo, C. M., McGlashan, T. H., & Morey, L. C. (2004). Childhood maltreatment associated with adult personality disorders: Findings from the collaborative longitudinal personality disorders study. *Journal of Personality Disorders*.
39. Biskin, R. S. (2015). The lifetime course of borderline personality disorder. *The Canadian Journal of Psychiatry*; Bateman, A. (2006). Psychoanalytic treatment of borderline personality disorder. *Psychiatric Times*.
40. Chapman, A. L. & Gratz, K. L. (2007). *The Borderline Personality Disorder Survival Guide.* New Harbinger Publications.
41. Bellis, M. A., Hughes, K., Leckenby, N., Hardcastle, K. A., Perkins, C., & Lowey, H. (2014). Measuring mortality and the burden of adult disease associated with adverse childhood experiences in England: A national survey. *Journal of Public Health*; Merrick, M. T., Ford, D. C., Ports, K. A., Guinn, A. S., Chen, J., Klevens, J., Metzler, M., Jones, C. M., Simon, T. R., Daniel, V. M., Ottley, P., & Mercy, J. A. (2019). Vital signs: Estimated proportion of adult health problems attributable to adverse childhood experiences and implications for prevention – 25 states, 2015–2017. *Morbidity and Mortality Weekly Report*.
42. Cichowski, S. B., Rogers, R. G., Clark, E. A., Murata, E., Murata, A.,

& Murata, G. (2017). Military sexual trauma in female veterans is associated with chronic pain conditions. *Military Medicine*.
43. Moussaoui, D. & Grover, S. R. (2022). The association between childhood adversity and risk of dysmenorrhea, pelvic pain, and dyspareunia in adolescents and young adults: A systematic review. *Journal of Pediatric and Adolescent Gynecology*; Bertone-Johnson, E. R., Whitcomb, B. W., Missmer, S. A., Manson, J. E., Hankinson, S. E., & Rich-Edwards, J. W. (2014). Early life emotional, physical, and sexual abuse and the development of premenstrual syndrome: A longitudinal study. *Journal of Women's Health*; Wittchen, H. U., Perkonigg, A., & Pfister, H. (2003). Trauma and PTSD: An overlooked pathogenic pathway for premenstrual dysphoric disorder? *Archives of Women's Mental Health*; Morishita, C., Inoue, T., Honyashiki, M., Ono, M., Iwata, Y., Tanabe, H., Kusumi, I., & Masuya, J. (2022). Roles of childhood maltreatment, personality traits, and life stress in the prediction of severe premenstrual symptoms. *BioPsychoSocial Medicine*; Faleschini, S., Tiemeier, H., Rifas-Shiman, S. L., Rich-Edwards, J., Joffe, H., Perng, W., Shifren, J., Chavarro, J. E., Hivert, M.-F., & Oken, E. (2022). Longitudinal associations of psychosocial stressors with menopausal symptoms and well-being among women in midlife. *Menopause*; Yang, Q., Þórðardóttir, E. B., Hauksdóttir, A., Aspelund, T., Jakobsdóttir, J., Halldorsdottir, T., Tomasson, G., Rúnarsdóttir, H., Danielsdottir, H. B., Bertone-Johnson, E. R., Sjölander, A., Fang, F., Lu, D., & Valdimarsdóttir, U. A. (2022). Association between adverse childhood experiences and premenstrual disorders: A cross-sectional analysis of 11,973 women. *BMC Medicine*.
44. Cadman, L., Waller, J., Ashdown-Barr, L., & Szarewski, A. (2012). Barriers to cervical screening in women who have experienced sexual abuse: An exploratory study: Table 1. *Journal of Family Planning and Reproductive Health Care*.
45. Yepez, D., Grandes, X. A., Talanki Manjunatha, R., Habib, S., & Sangaraju, S. L. (2022). Fibromyalgia and depression: A literature review of their shared aspects. *Cureus*; Ionescu, C.-E., Popescu, C. C., Agache, M., Dinache, G., & Codreanu, C. (2022). Depression in rheumatoid arthritis: A narrative review–diagnostic challenges, pathogenic mechanisms and effects. *Medicina*; Jahangir, S., Adjepong, D., Al-Shami, H. A., & Malik, B. H. (2020). Is there an association between migraine and major depressive disorder?

A narrative review. *Cureus*; Anxiety & Depression Association of America (2022). The relationship between migraines and depression. adaa.org.

46. Van der Kolk, B. (2014). *The Body Keeps the Score*. Penguin Books.
47. Song, H., Fang, F., Tomasson, G., Arnberg, F. K., Mataix-Cols, D., Fernández de la Cruz, L., Almqvist, C., Fall, K., & Valdimarsdóttir, U. A. (2018). Association of stress-related disorders with subsequent autoimmune disease. *JAMA*.
48. Angum, F., Khan, T., Kaler, J., Siddiqui, L., & Hussain, A. (2020). The prevalence of autoimmune disorders in women: A narrative review. *Cureus*; National Center for PTSD (2023). How common is PTSD in adults? US Department of Veteran Affairs. ptsd.va.gov.
49. Shors, T. J., Tobón, K., DiFeo, G., Durham, D. M., & Chang, H. Y. M. (2016). Sexual Conspecific Aggressive Response (SCAR): A model of sexual trauma that disrupts maternal learning and plasticity in the female brain. *Scientific Reports*.
50. Shors, T. J. & Millon, E. M. (2016). Sexual trauma and the female brain. *Frontiers in Neuroendocrinology*; Schoenfeld, T. J. & Gould, E. (2012). Stress, stress hormones, and adult neurogenesis. *Experimental Neurology*.
51. I'm speculating, but there is a connection between the jaw and pelvic floor. Giles, J. (2023). If you're a jaw clencher, there's a good chance your pelvic floor is also too tight. *Well+Good*.

Chapter 9 Sexy But Not Sexual

1. Grigoriadis, V. (2003). Princess Paris. *Rolling Stone*.
2. Smith, K. (2005). The inescapable Paris. *Vanity Fair*.
3. Weiss, S. (2022). Pubic hair and public norms: How beauty brands are navigating changing personal grooming attitudes and practices. *Beauty Independent*.
4. O'Regan, K. (2013). Labiaplasty, Part I. *Guernica*; Reuters (2012). Timeline: A short history of breast implants. Reuters.com.
5. Davey, M. (2022). Johnson & Johnson reaches $300m settlement over pelvic mesh implants. *The Guardian*; Knaus, C. (2017). Pelvic mesh victims disgusted at suggestion of anal sex as solution. *The Guardian*.
6. Jo's Cervical Cancer Trust (2019). Not so simple: The impact of cervical cell changes and treatment. jostrust.org.
7. The authors conclude that "the LEEP procedure itself appears to

have a minimal, if any, clinically important adverse effect on sexual function" – yet it's hard to imagine any loss of sexual function feeling "minimal" to the patient. While some patients get back to their usual sex lives with no trouble, there is also a documented sub-population with significant and lasting side effects. Inna, N., Phianmongkhol, Y., & Charoenkwan, K. (2010). Sexual function after loop electrosurgical excision procedure for cervical dysplasia. *Journal of Sexual Medicine*; Giovannetti, O., Tomalty, D., Greco, S., & Adams, M. (2022). Self-report assessment of sexual function after LEEP in women who report negative outcomes. *Journal of Sexual Medicine*.

8. Smothers, H. (2019). This routine gyno procedure could mean you never orgasm again. *Cosmopolitan*; Giovannetti, O., Tomalty, D., Greco, S., Kment, B., Komisaruk, B., Hannan, J., Goldstein, S., Goldstein, I., & Adams, M. A. (2023). Patient and provider perspectives on LEEP/LLETZ treatment and outcomes: An interview study. *Journal of Sexual Medicine*.

9. Sklavos, M. M., Spracklen, C. N., Saftlas, A. F., & Pinto, L. A. (2014). Does loop electrosurgical excision procedure of the uterine cervix affect anti-Müllerian hormone levels? *BioMed Research International*.

10. Komisaruk, B. & Del Cerro, M. C. (2020). The cervix is sensitive, and surgeons need to acknowledge the part it plays in some women's pleasure. *The Conversation*.

11. Petitti, D. (2005). Four decades of research on hormonal contraception. *Permanente Journal*.

12. Daniels, K., Mosher, W. D., & Jones, J. (2013). Contraceptive methods women have ever used: United States, 1982–2010. *National Statistics Reports*.

13. Goldstein, A., Pukall, C. F., & Goldstein, I. (2011). *When Sex Hurts*. Da Capo Lifelong; Battaglia, C., Morotti, E., Persico, N., Battaglia, B., Busacchi, P., Casadio, P., Paradisi, R., & Venturoli, S. (2014). Clitoral vascularization and sexual behavior in young patients treated with drospirenone-ethinyl estradiol or contraceptive vaginal ring: A prospective, randomized, pilot study. *Journal of Sexual Medicine*.

14. Zethraeus, N., Dreber, A., Ranehill, E., Blomberg, L., Labrie, F., von Schoultz, B., Johannesson, M., & Hirschberg, A. L. (2016). Combined oral contraceptives and sexual function in women – A double-blind, randomized, placebo-controlled trial. *Journal of Clinical Endocrinology & Metabolism*.

15. Aponte, M. et al. (2013). Incidence of pelvic pain symptoms in community-dwelling young women and relationship to use and type of oral contraceptive pills. 108th Annual Meeting of the American Urological Association.
16. Smith, N. K., Jozkowski, K. N., & Sanders, S. A. (2014). Hormonal contraception and female pain, orgasm and sexual pleasure. *Journal of Sexual Medicine.*
17. MacMillan, C. (2024). What women should know about intrauterine devices (IUDs). Yale Medicine. yalemedicine.org.
18. Casado-Espada, N. M., de Alarcón, R., de la Iglesia-Larrad, J. I., Bote-Bonaechea, B., & Montejo, Á. L. (2019). Hormonal contraceptives, female sexual dysfunction, and managing strategies: A review. *Journal of Clinical Medicine.*
19. Littlejohn, K. (2021). *Just Get on the Pill.* University of California Press.
20. Planned Parenthood (2024). What are the disadvantages of the pull out method? plannedparenthood.org.
21. Some clinicians have observed smaller clitorises and less labial development in women who started hormonal birth control as teens. Casperson, K. (Host). (2023). When Sex Hurts [Podcast episode]. *You Are Not Broken.*
22. Brody, D. and Gu, Q. (2020). Antidepressant use among adults: United States, 2015–2018. National Center for Health Statistics. cdc.gov; Lorenz, T., Rullo, J., & Faubion, S. (2016). Antidepressant-induced female sexual dysfunction. *Mayo Clinic Proceedings.*
23. Armstrong, E. A., England, P., & Fogarty, A. C. K. (2012). Accounting for women's orgasm and sexual enjoyment in college hookups and relationships. *American Sociological Review.*
24. Séguin, L. J., Rodrigue, C., & Lavigne, J. (2017). Consuming ecstasy: Representations of male and female orgasm in mainstream pornography. *Journal of Sex Research.*
25. Harvey-Jenner, C. (2015). The orgasm gap is REAL – Women are losing out. *Cosmopolitan.*
26. Grajek, M., Krupa-Kotara, K., Grot, M., Kujawińska, M., Helisz, P., Gwioździk, W., Białek-Dratwa, A., Staśkiewicz, W., & Kobza, J. (2022). Perception of the body image in women after childbirth and the specific determinants of their eating behavior: Cross-sectional study (Silesia, Poland). *International Journal of Environmental Research and Public Health.*
27. Kingsberg, S. & Millheiser, L. (2016). Mature women's attitudes

about the impact of sexual concerns on relationship and sexual satisfaction. North American Menopause Society (NAMS) 2016 Annual Meeting.
28. See chapter 3, n. 33.
29. Thomas, H. N., Hamm, M., Hess, R., & Thurston, R. C. (2018). Changes in sexual function among midlife women. *Menopause*; Forbes, M. K., Eaton, N. R., & Krueger, R. F. (2016). Sexual quality of life and aging: A prospective study of a nationally representative sample. *Journal of Sex Research*.

Chapter 10 Womanhood Is Not an Illness
1. See chapter 2, n. 25.
2. Weiss, S. (2019). Experts say Lyme disease can cause this bladder issue. *Bustle*.
3. Part of the confusion is that some distinguish between "classic" IC, with visible lesions on the bladder, and IC symptoms caused by something else. This may be a false dichotomy because infections can cause lesions, as they did for America. Still, I am by no means implying *everyone* can cure their IC this instant or they've failed. I *am* hopeful more people will be able to once the many causes become clearer and easier to diagnose. Weiss, S. (2019). What causes interstitial cystitis? How 10 women got to the root of their bladder pain. *Bustle*.
4. Mayo Clinic (2023). Vulvodynia. mayoclinic.org.
5. Kesavelu, D. & Jog, P. (2023). Current understanding of antibiotic-associated dysbiosis and approaches for its management. *Therapeutic Advances in Infectious Disease*; Sánchez-Pérez, S., Comas-Basté, O., Duelo, A., Veciana-Nogués, M. T., Berlanga, M., Latorre-Moratalla, M. L., & Vidal-Carou, M. C. (2022). Intestinal dysbiosis in patients with histamine intolerance. *Nutrients*; Harlow, B. L., He, W., & Nguyen, R. H. N. (2009). Allergic reactions and risk of vulvodynia. *Annals of Epidemiology*; Rosa, A. C. & Fantozzi, R. (2013). The role of histamine in neurogenic inflammation. *British Journal of Pharmacology*.
6. Gangi, S. & Johansson, O. (2000). A theoretical model based upon mast cells and histamine to explain the recently proclaimed sensitivity to electric and/or magnetic fields in humans. *Medical Hypotheses*; Cirino, E. (2023). Should you be worried about EMF exposure? *Healthline*; Bell, S. & Newson, L. (2021). Histamine

intolerance (HIT). Balance. balance-menopause.com; Nowak, K., Jabłońska, E., & Ratajczak-Wrona, W. (2019). Immunomodulatory effects of synthetic endocrine disrupting chemicals on the development and functions of human immune cells. *Environment International*; Shah, S. (2012). Hormonal link to autoimmune allergies. *ISRN Allergy*; Bonds, R. S. & Midoro-Horiuti, T. (2013). Estrogen effects in allergy and asthma. *Current Opinion in Allergy & Clinical Immunology*.
7. Wantke, F., Götz, M., & Jarisch, R. (1994). The red wine provocation test: Intolerance to histamine as a model for food intolerance. *Allergy and Asthma Proceedings*.
8. Cleveland Clinic (2024). Dysbiosis. my.clevelandclinic.org.
9. Ramey, see Part 1, n. 2; Eller-Smith, O. C., Nicol, A. L., & Christianson, J. A. (2018). Potential mechanisms underlying centralized pain and emerging therapeutic interventions. *Frontiers in Cellular Neuroscience*.
10. As sex-positive reverend Beverly Dale told me: "The liberating ideas of Jesus and the egalitarian principles of the early church ultimately became blips on the screen of history" in the wake of Romanized Christian leadership.

Chapter 11 Period Pleasure

1. Anca, R. (2024). Can you really reach orgasm using just the power of your mind? *Men's Health*.
2. Goldhill, O. (2016). Period pain can be "almost as bad as a heart attack." Why aren't we researching how to treat it? *Quartz*; Baxter-Wright, D. (2016). Expert say period pains can be "as bad as having a heart attack." *Cosmopolitan*; Driver, G. (2018). Doctors have finally ruled menstrual cramps are as painful as heart attacks. *Marie Claire*.
3. Driver, G. (2018). Doctors have finally ruled menstrual cramps are as painful as heart attacks. *Elle*.
4. MTV UK (2019). Guys try period pain! MTV Style. youtube.com.
5. Maybury, K. (2013). A positive approach to menarche and menstruation. American Psychological Association. apadivisions.org; University College London (2024). Women's mental agility is better when they're on their period, study finds. *Science Daily*; Fahs, B. (2020). There will be blood: Women's positive and negative experiences with menstruation. *Women's Reproductive Health*.

6. Carter, K., Bassis, C., McKee, K., Bullock, K., Eastman, A., Young, V., & Bell, J. (2018). The impact of tampon use on the vaginal microbiota across four menstrual cycles. *American Journal of Obstetrics and Gynecology*; University of Texas at Austin (2019). Period products: The good, the bad, and the ugly. uthealthaustin.org; Cleveland Clinic (2022). Toxic shock syndrome. my.clevelandclinic.org; Taylor, M. (2015). 7 great things that happen when you stop using tampons. *Prevention*.
7. Shearston, J. A., Upson, K., Gordon, M., Do, V., Balac, O., Nguyen, K., Yan, B., Kioumourtzoglou, M., & Schilling, K. (2024). Tampons as a source of exposure to metal(loid)s. *Environment International*; Bobei, T. I. (2023). The relationship between lifestyle, medical history and the presence of dysmenorrhea. *Romanian Journal of Clinical Research*.
8. Valiani, M., Ghasemi, N., Bahadoran, P., & Heshmat, R. (2024). The effects of massage therapy on dysmenorrhea caused by endometriosis. *Iranian Journal of Nursing and Midwifery Research*; Mirabi, P., Alamolhoda, S. H., Esmaeilzadeh, S., & Mojab, F. (2014). Effect of medicinal herbs on primary dysmenorrhoea: A systematic review. *Iranian Journal of Pharmaceutical Research*; Sharghi, M., Mansurkhani, S. M., Ashtary-Larky, D., Kooti, W., Niksefat, M., Firoozbakht, M., Behzadifar, M., Azami, M., Servatyari, K., & Jouybari, L. (2019). An update and systematic review on the treatment of primary dysmenorrhea. *JBRA Assisted Reproduction*; Guo, Y., Liu, F.-Y., Shen, Y., Xu, J.-Y., Xie, L.-Z., Li, S.-Y., Ding, D.-N., Zhang, D.-Q., & Han, F.-J. (2021). Complementary and alternative medicine for dysmenorrhea caused by endometriosis: A review of utilization and mechanism. *Evidence-Based Complementary and Alternative Medicine*; Mount Sinai (2024). Menstrual pain. mountsinai.org; Muraskin, A. (2013). Can abdominal massage help painful menstruation? Side Effects Public Media; University of Utah (2017). Natural remedies for period pains. healthcare.utah.edu.
9. Brabaw, K. (2023). So that's why you get so horny during your period. *Refinery29*; Weiss, S. (2019). The real reason you get horny during your period. *Bustle*.
10. Knight, J. (2016). *The Complete Guide to Fertility Awareness*. Routledge; Weschler, T. (2015). *Taking Charge of Your Fertility*. William Morrow; Billings, E. L. (2024). The simplicity of the

ovulation method and its application in various circumstances. *Acta Europaea Fertilitatis*; Learn Body Literacy (2024). The 3 primary fertility signs. learnbodyliteracy.com.
11. Hickey, M., Hunter, M. S., Santoro, N., & Ussher, J. (2022). Normalising menopause. *BMJ*.
12. Nosek, M., Kennedy, H. P., Beyene, Y., Taylor, D., Gilliss, C., & Lee, K. (2010). The effects of perceived stress and attitudes toward menopause and aging on symptoms of menopause. *Journal of Midwifery & Women's Health*; Im, E.-O., Lee, S. H., & Chee, W. (2010). Subethnic differences in the menopausal symptom experience of Asian American midlife women. *Journal of Transcultural Nursing*.
13. Harlow, S. D., Burnett-Bowie, S.-A. M., Greendale, G. A., Avis, N. E., Reeves, A. N., Richards, T. R., & Lewis, T. T. (2022). Disparities in reproductive aging and midlife health between black and white women: The Study of Women's Health Across the Nation (SWAN). *Women's Midlife Health*.
14. Jamali, S., Javadpour, S., Mosalanejad, L., & Parnian, R. (2016). Attitudes about sexual activity among postmenopausal women in different ethnic groups: A cross-sectional study in Jahrom, Iran. *Journal of Reproduction & Infertility*; Hickey, M., LaCroix, A. Z., Doust, J., Mishra, G. D., Sivakami, M., Garlick, D., & Hunter, M. S. (2024). An empowerment model for managing menopause. *The Lancet*; Upham, B. (2023). 6 unexpected benefits you'll be happy to know about menopause. *Everyday Health*.

Chapter 12 No Pleasure, No Gain
1. Basanta, S. & Nuño de la Rosa, L. (2022). The female orgasm and the homology concept in evolutionary biology. *Journal of Morphology*.
2. Knöfel Magnusson, A. (2009). My corona: The hymen and the myths that surround it. *Scarleteen*; Our Bodies Ourselves (2021). What exactly is a hymen? ourbodiesourselves.com.
3. Valenti, J. (2009). *The Purity Myth*. Seal Press.
4. Staniforth, J. (2021). Should we re-brand virginity? *BBC*.
5. @thought_bug_ (2019). "Losing/taking virginity..." X. x.com/thought_bug_/status/1191326530250653697.
6. Go Ask Alice (2015). Can I stretch my hymen? goaskalice.columbia.edu.

Chapter 13 In Joy Thou Shalt Bring Forth Children
1. Postel, T. (2013). Childbirth climax: The revealing of obstetrical orgasm. *Sexologies*.
2. Gaskin, I. M. (2003). *Ina May's Guide to Childbirth*. Bantam Books.
3. Haelle, T. (2020). What is a doula? And do you need one? *The New York Times*; Murphy, C. (2018). Midwives are growing in popularity. Here's what you need to know. *Healthline*; US Government Accountability Office (2023). Midwives: Information on births, workforce, and midwifery education. gao.gov.
4. National Partnership for Women & Families (2018). Continuous support for women during childbirth: 2017 Cochrane Review update key takeaways. *Journal of Perinatal Education*.
5. Stone, S. (nd). Shalome's rockstar orgasmic birth experience. orgasmicbirth.com.
6. Tabib, M., Humphrey, T., Forbes-McKay, K., & Lau, A. (2021). Expectant parents' perspectives on the influence of a single antenatal relaxation class: A qualitative study. *Complementary Therapies in Clinical Practice*.
7. Elvander, C., Cnattingius, S., & Kjerulff, K. H. (2013). Birth experience in women with low, intermediate or high levels of fear: Findings from the first baby study. *Birth*.
8. Marie, S. (2021). Orgasmic labor and birth: Could it be for you? *Healthline*; Morhenn, V., Beavin, L. E., & Zak, P. J. (2012). Massage increases oxytocin and reduces adrenocorticotropin hormone in humans. *Alternative Therapies in Health and Medicine*; Frey Law, L. A., Evans, S., Knudtson, J., Nus, S., Scholl, K., & Sluka, K. A. (2008). Massage reduces pain perception and hyperalgesia in experimental muscle pain: A randomized, controlled trial. *Journal of Pain*; Gay, C., Alappattu, M. J., Coronado, R. A., Horn, M. E., & Bishop, M. D. (2013). Effect of a single session of muscle-biased therapy on pain sensitivity: A systematic review and meta-analysis of randomized controlled trials. *Journal of Pain Research*.
9. Fields, H. L. (2018). How expectations influence pain. *PAIN*; Hughes, M. (2024). Why you need to relax your pelvic floor during birth (and how to do it). drmaehughes.com; Physiopedia (2018). Childbirth and the pelvic floor. physiopedia.com.
10. According to endocrinologist Aimee Eyvazzadeh, severe cold can lead to constriction of blood vessels and oxygen deprivation for the baby.

11. Asherah is a mother goddess from the Canaanite religion.
12. As with PMS, hormones may contribute to postpartum depression but are not typically the root cause, says King. Agrawal, I., Mehendale, A. M., & Malhotra, R. (2022). Risk factors of postpartum depression. *Cureus*; Schiller, C. E., Meltzer-Brody, S., Rubinow, D. R. (2014). The role of reproductive hormones in postpartum depression. *CNS Spectrums*.
13. Weiss, S. (2022). Sex after birth: How does it affect orgasms? *Dame*.

Chapter 14 I Will Greatly Multiply Thy Orgasms
1. Sophia Wallace (2024). "Clit Rodeo." sophiawallace.art; Mosbergen, D. (2013). Cliteracy 101: Artist Sophia Wallace wants you to know the truth about the clitoris. *The Huffington Post*.
2. @sekswijzer (2022). "By Sophia Wallace..." Instagram. instagram.com/sekswijzer/p/ClWGpI8oz41.
3. Riley, A. J. & Riley, E. J. (1978). A controlled study to evaluate directed masturbation in the management of primary orgasmic failure in women. *British Journal of Psychiatry*.
4. If antidepressants are hindering your sex life, speak to a psychiatrist about a plan to taper off and/or try a new medication.
5. Solot & Miller, see chapter 5, n. 18.
6. Rowland, D. L., Cempel, L. M., & Tempel, A. R. (2018). Women's attributions regarding why they have difficulty reaching orgasm. *Journal of Sex & Marital Therapy*.
7. I don't necessarily agree that women are more orgasmic. I think we're all infinitely orgasmic.

Chapter 15 Living Life Orgasmically
1. A few small studies support the use of escharotic treatments, though they are not yet widely researched or recommended. Windstar, K., Dunlap, C., & Zwickey, H. (2014). Escharotic treatment for ECC-positive CIN3 in childbearing years: A case report. *Integrative Medicine: A Clinician's Journal*; Hudson, T. S. (1991). Consecutive case study research of carcinoma *in situ* of cervix employing local escharotic treatment combined with nutritional therapy. *Journal of Naturopathic Medicine*; Hudson, T. S. (1993). Escharotic treatment for cervical dysplasia and carcinoma. *Journal of Naturopathic Medicine*.
2. Turner, K. (2015). *Radical Remission*. HarperOne.
3. See, for instance, the coital alignment technique: Lehmiller, J.

(2019). This sex position increases the odds of simultaneous orgasm for men and women. sexandpsychology.com.
4. See Introduction, n. 3, and chapter 5, n. 34.
5. Cleveland Clinic (2022). Clitoris. my.clevelandclinic.org; Whipple, B. & Komisaruk, B. R. (2022). Brain (PET) responses to vaginal-cervical self-stimulation in women with complete spinal cord injury: Preliminary findings. *Journal of Sex & Marital Therapy*; Komisaruk, B. R., Whipple, B., Crawford, A., Grimes, S., Liu, W.-C., Kalnin, A., & Mosier, K. (2004). Brain activation during vaginocervical self-stimulation and orgasm in women with complete spinal cord injury: fMRI evidence of mediation by the vagus nerves. *Brain Research*; Pfaus, J. G., Quintana, G. R., Mac Cionnaith, C., & Parada, M. (2016). The whole versus the sum of some of the parts: Toward resolving the apparent controversy of clitoral versus vaginal orgasms. *Socioaffective Neuroscience & Psychology*.
6. Weitkamp, K. & Wehrli, V. (2023). Women's experiences of different types of orgasms – A call for pleasure literacy? *International Journal of Sexual Health*.
7. I say "healthy" because this data excludes those with hysterectomies and uterine fibroids. Interestingly, those with fibroids reported more orgasms from cervical and vaginal stimulation. Cutler, W. B., McCoy, N. L., Zacher, M. G., Genovese, E., & Friedman, E. (2000). Sexual response in women. American College of Obstetricians and Gynecologists 2000 meeting.
8. Younis, I., Fattah, M., & Maamoun, M. (2016). Female hot spots: Extragenital erogenous zones. *Human Andrology*; Herbenick, D. (2015). *The Coregasm Workout*. Seal Press; Tee-Melegrito, R. A. (2022). What is a coregasm and how do people achieve them? *Medical News Today*; Pfaus, J. G. & Tsarski, K. (2022). A case of female orgasm without genital stimulation. *Sexual Medicine*; Whipple, B., Ogden, G., & Komisaruk, B. R. (1992). Physiological correlates of imagery-induced orgasm in women. *Archives of Sexual Behavior*; Leavitt, L. (2009). Scientists study mental orgasms through MRIs. *TechCrunch*.
9. Kratochvíl, S. (1993). Multiple orgasms in women. *Ceskoslovenska Psychiatrie*; Darling, C. A., Davidson, J. K., & Jennings, D. A. (1991). The female sexual response revisited: Understanding the multiorgasmic experience in women. *Archives of Sexual Behavior*.
10. Davison, S. L., Bell, R. J., LaChina, M., Holden, S. L., & Davis, S. R.

(2009). The relationship between self-reported sexual satisfaction and general well-being in women. *Journal of Sexual Medicine*; Kashdan, T. B., Goodman, F. R., Stiksma, M., Milius, C. R., & McKnight, P. E. (2018). Sexuality leads to boosts in mood and meaning in life with no evidence for the reverse direction: A daily diary investigation. *Emotion*.

11. Brennan, D. (2021). What to know about oxytocin hormone. *WebMD*; Cleveland Clinic (2022). Orgasm. my.clevelandclinic.org; Mitrokostas, S. (2019). Here's what happens to your body and brain when you orgasm. *ScienceAlert*.
12. To be clear, though, I usually prefer combining penetration with clitoral stimulation and have no qualms about that.
13. Shah, D. T., Glover, D. D., & Larsen, B. (1995). In situ mycotoxin production by Candida albicans in women with vaginitis. *Gynecologic and Obstetric Investigation*; Coda, L., Cassis, P., Angioletti, S., Angeloni, C., Piloni, S., & Testa, C. (2021). Evaluation of gut microbiota in patients with vulvovestibular syndrome. *Journal of Clinical Medicine Research*.

Epilogue: Original Virtue

1. That's not his real name, by the way ... I won't kiss and tell ;)
2. Gitz-Johansen, T. (2020). Jung and the spirit: A review of Jung's discussions of the phenomenon of spirit. *Journal of Analytical Psychology*; *Holy Bible: King James Version* (2017). Genesis 2:7. Green World Classics.